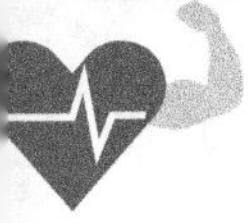

# Quick Workout for Seniors Age 60+

## Simple Exercise and Stretching Positions for Strength Training, Flexibility, Mobility, and Cardio - An Illustrated Guide

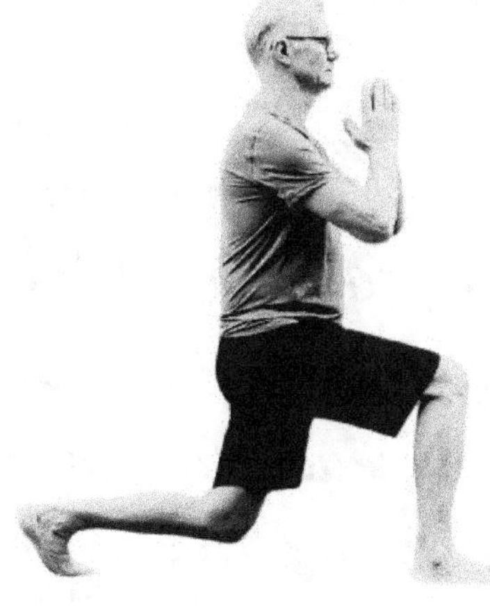

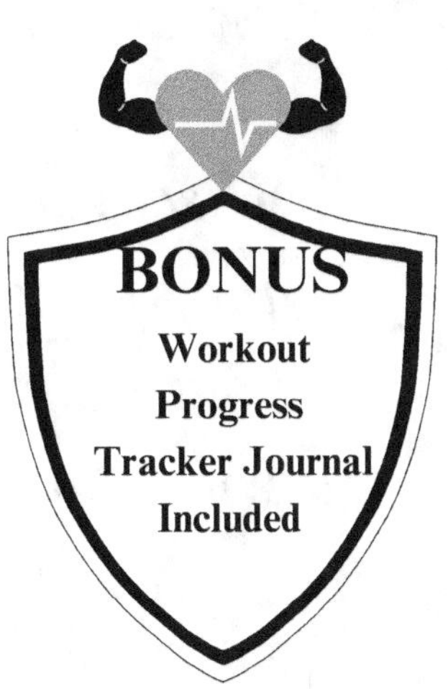


By Desmond T. Hall

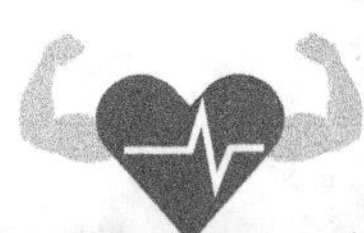

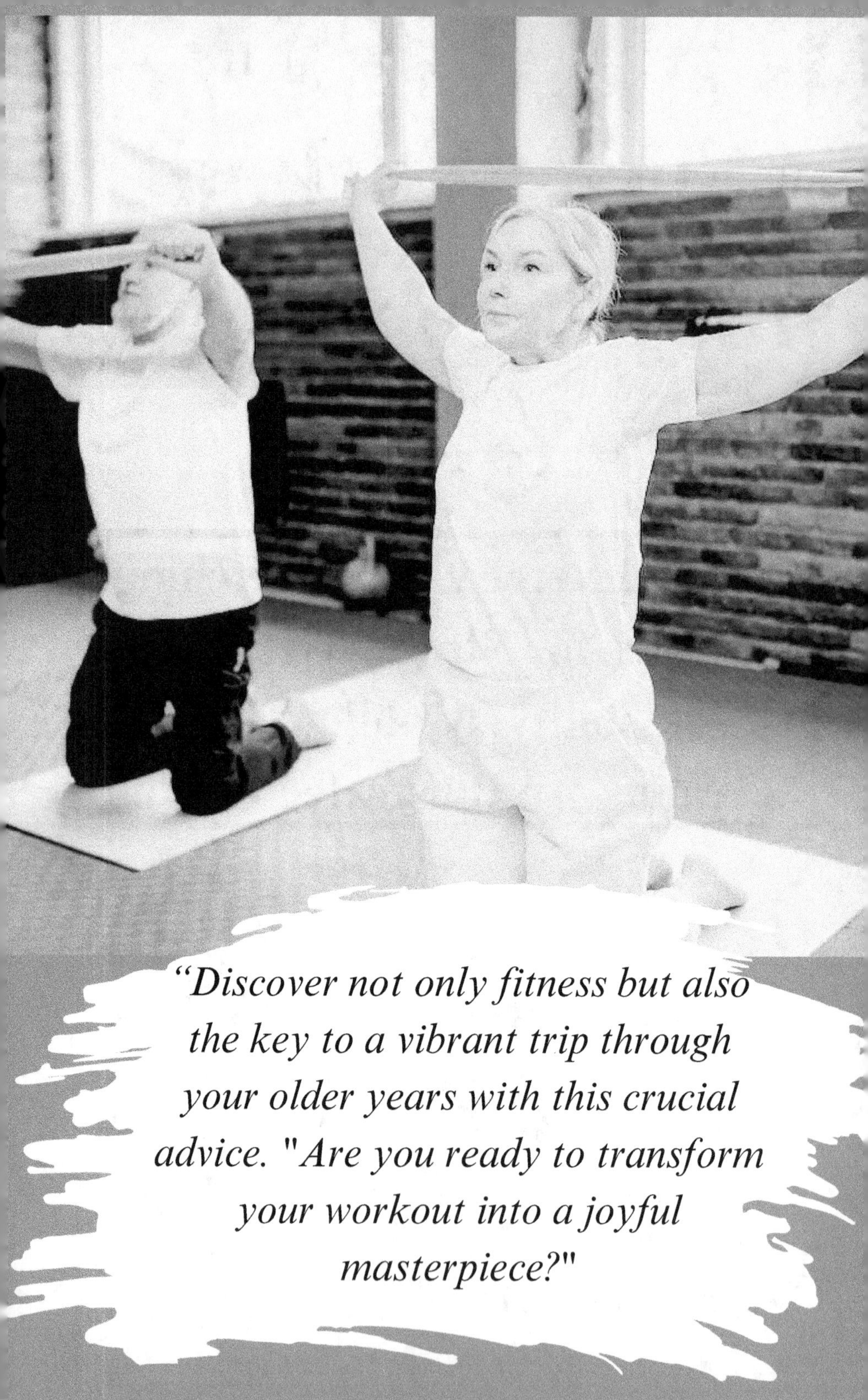
"Discover not only fitness but also the key to a vibrant trip through your older years with this crucial advice. "Are you ready to transform your workout into a joyful masterpiece?"

# Copyright © 2023 by Desmond T. Hall



# Disclaimer ⚠

This book is a work of nonfiction. Names, characters, places, and incidents are either the product of the author's imagination or are used fictitiously. Any resemblance to actual persons, living or dead, business establishments, events, or locales is entirely coincidental.

# WHAT YOU WILL GET IN THIS BOOK

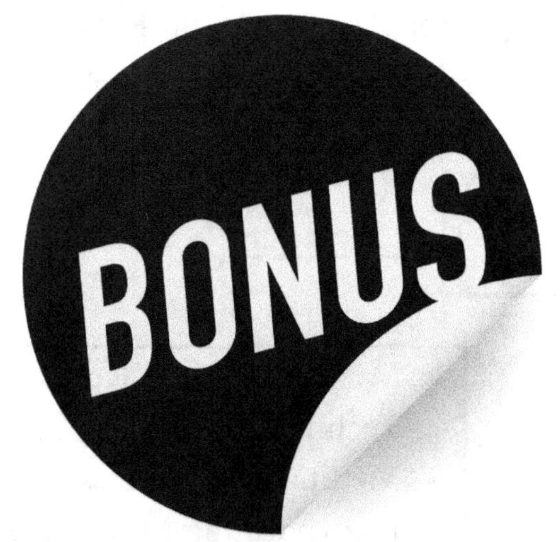


# Progress Tracker
# Journal

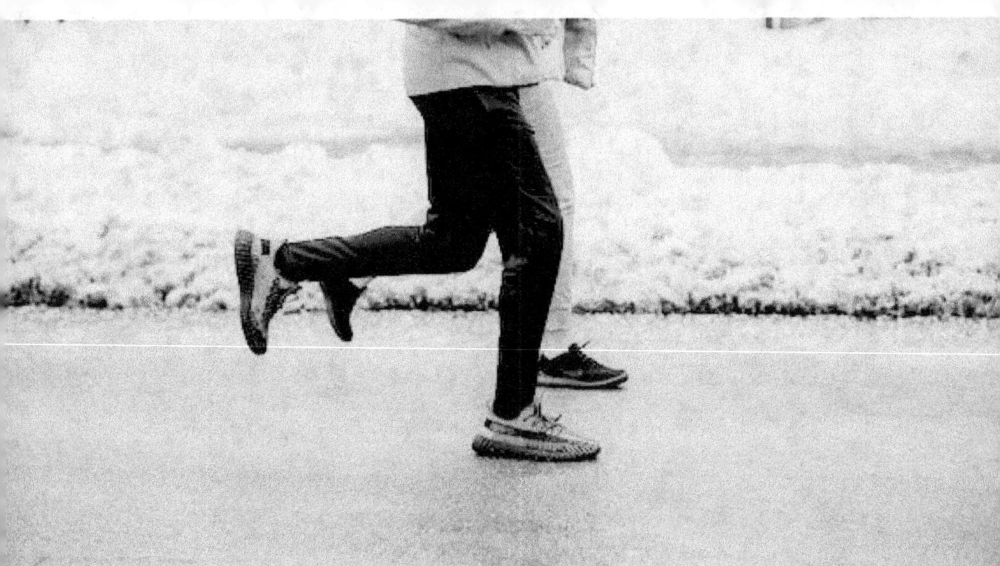

# INTRODUCTION

With 'Quick Workout for Seniors Age 60+,' you can enter a world where age is no barrier and energy knows no limitations. This book shines as a beacon of transformation in the quiet moments of realizing leg weakness or the subtle recognition of muscles asking for attention. Consider this: a robust life enhanced by strength, flexibility, and increased mobility. The discomfort of inactivity becomes more obvious as we age, and 'Quick Workout for Seniors' is the solution. It's a journey, not simply via exercises, but into a life free of the constraints we frequently accept. Discover the ability to defy aging one easy but powerful workout at a time. Within these pages is a guide to a pain-free, exciting chapter of your life. Allow the metamorphosis to begin.

## *Let's get Started!*

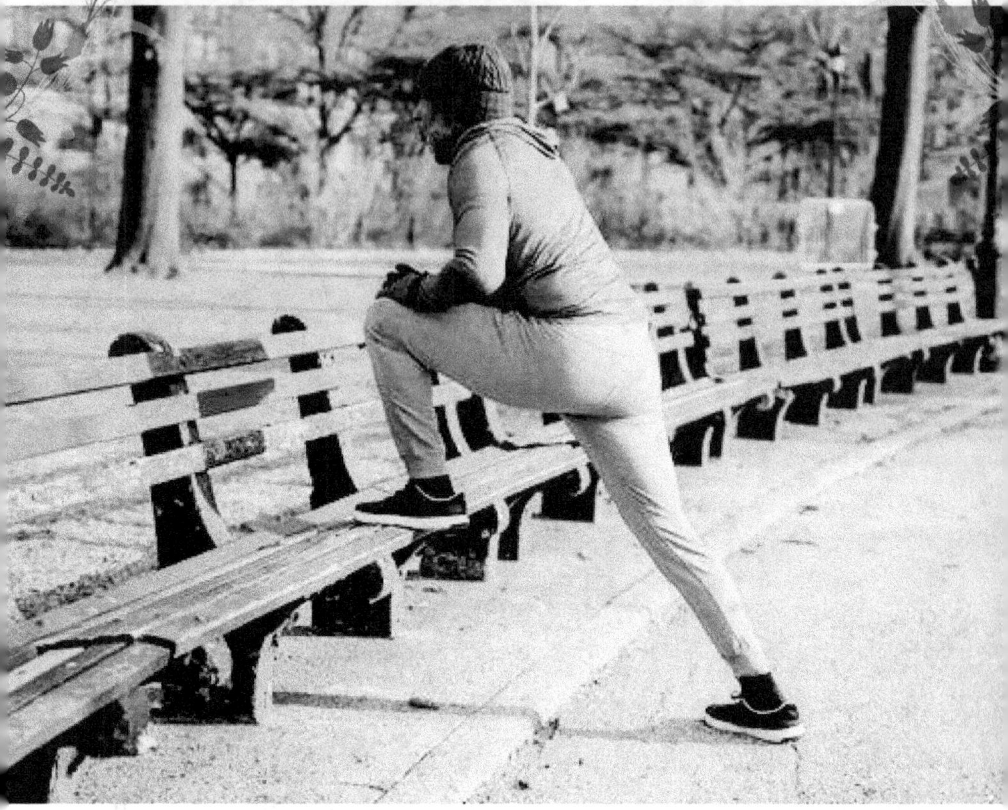

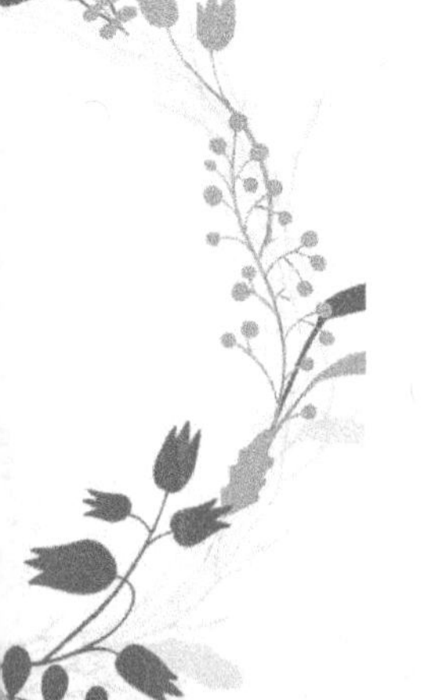

> **"The Goal here is not to "feel the burn," but rather to softly wake up your muscles."**

# CHAPTER 1

## Understanding Senior Fitness

The Quick Workout for Seniors Over 60 has several advantages, including a specialized approach to health and vitality at this specific stage of life. For starters, it improves flexibility and range of motion. Joints might tighten and muscles can lose pliability as we age. This gentle workout leads elders through stretches and motions meant to restore and increase flexibility, allowing for more ease in daily tasks.

Balance and stability are critical, and this workout emphasizes them specifically. Seniors who engage in exercises that test their balance strengthen their core strength and lower their chance of falling, promoting a better sense of confidence and independence.

Strength exercise, however light and simple, is an essential component. It prevents muscle atrophy, which is normal with aging and promotes functional strength for daily duties. These workouts improve total muscle tone, which contributes to a strong and sturdy body.

Mindfulness is weaved throughout the book, promoting mental clarity and a stronger mind-body connection. Seniors can achieve a state of presence via focused breathing and deliberate movement, which relieves tension and promotes a sense of serenity.

Finally, this workout fosters a long-term pattern by fostering discipline and consistency. It encourages elders to establish realistic fitness objectives and alter their routines as needed, promoting a lifelong commitment to their health and well-being. In essence, the advantages of this short workout for seniors over 60 go well beyond the physical, touching on every aspect of living a vital, meaningful life.

## Cultivating a Positive Mindset

Seniors who wish to retain their physical health and independence must cultivate a positive outlook. Here are a few tips for creating a pleasant attitude during a brief exercise for elders over 60.

- **Create reasonable objectives for your exercise program:** Seniors should create realistic goals for their exercise program, such as walking 30 minutes each day or practicing strength training exercises twice a week. They should also keep track of their development and recognize their accomplishments along the road.
- **Find fun activities:** Seniors should engage in enjoyable hobbies such as dance, swimming, or gardening. Seniors may keep motivated and interested in their training program by selecting things that they like.
- **Stay sociable:** Seniors should maintain their social lives by exercising with friends or enrolling in a fitness class. Seniors who socialize may remain

motivated and devoted to their training program.

- Seniors may practice mindfulness throughout their exercise by concentrating on their breath and being present in the moment. This may assist seniors in reducing stress and anxiety while also improving their general well-being.
- utilize positive self-talk: During an exercise, seniors should utilize positive self-talk such as "I am strong" or "I can do this." Seniors may enhance their confidence and motivation by employing positive self-talk.
- Small accomplishments should be celebrated by seniors, such as finishing an exercise or accomplishing a fitness goal. Small celebrations

## Safety and Precautions

As seniors begin their fitness journey, safety, and safeguards become the foundation of a successful and sustainable workout regimen. The aging body needs careful thought, and knowing how to handle possible hazards is critical. let us look into the main features of senior fitness safety and precautions, discussing the necessity of individualized routines, the relevance of medical consultations, and practical techniques for risk reduction.

- Understanding the Specific Requirements of Senior Fitness: Senior fitness involves a nuanced strategy that takes into account the unique needs of aging bodies.

Age-related physiological changes, such as decreased bone density, joint flexibility, and muscle mass, need a deliberate and careful approach to exercise.

- **Flexibility and joint health:** Seniors are more prone to stiffness and decreased flexibility. It is critical to do exercises that gradually enhance the range of motion without creating strain or damage.
- **Considerations for the Cardiovascular System:** because of age-related changes in the cardiovascular system, cardio workouts must be carefully chosen. It is critical to balance the requirement for heart-healthy activities and the risk of severe stress.
- **Concerns About Bone Density:** Fractures are more likely in those who have osteoporosis or have low bone density. To strengthen bones without causing injury, strength training and weight-bearing activities must be selected with caution.
- **The Function of Medical Consultations:** Before elders begin a new exercise regimen, they should check with healthcare specialists. A full awareness of a person's medical history, current ailments, and any possible contraindications is essential for developing a safe and efficient exercise regimen.
- **Comprehensive Health Examinations:** Medical specialists may undertake comprehensive exams, such as cardiovascular health checks, bone density scans, and joint health evaluations, to adapt exercise suggestions to specific requirements.

- **Recognizing Contradictions:** Certain medical issues or drugs may have an impact on the sorts of workouts that are appropriate for seniors. Identifying these inconsistencies ensures that fitness plans do not aggravate pre-existing health problems.
- **Healthcare Providers and Fitness Instructors Communicate:** It is critical to facilitate communication between healthcare doctors and exercise instructors. This collaborative approach guarantees that exercise plans are consistent with medical guidance and that they may be changed as required.
- **Gradual Progression is a practical strategy for ensuring safety:** Seniors should begin with activities that are appropriate for their present fitness level and work their way up. This method reduces the danger of overexertion or injury while enabling the body to adapt to new physical demands.
- **Warm-ups and cool-downs should be done correctly:** Elders must include proper warm-up and cool-down activities. These exercises help to prepare the body for exercise by increasing flexibility and decreasing the chance of strains or accidents
- **Nutrition and Hydration:** Staying hydrated is critical for seniors who participate in physical exercise. Proper nutrition, including a nutrient-dense diet, promotes energy levels and general well-being.

- **Appropriate Footwear and Equipment:** Wearing appropriate footwear with enough support and comfortable training clothing helps to safety. This is particularly critical during workouts to decrease the danger of falling and improve overall stability.
- **Supervision and clear instructions:** During exercises, seniors benefit from precise and simple instructions. Having a certified fitness teacher or a supportive workout partner also adds an added layer of supervision, ensuring that exercises are executed properly.
- **Health Check-Ins regularly:** Health exams and check-ins with healthcare specialists regularly assist in monitoring any changes in health conditions. These updates may be used to make changes to the workout regimen.
- **Paying Attention to the Body:** It is critical to encourage elders to pay attention to their bodies and disclose any discomfort or suffering. Potential injuries may be avoided by modifying or discontinuing a workout as necessary.
- **Adapting Exercises to Meet Individual Needs:** Every senior has a different health profile, and exercise programs should be adaptive to meet their specific demands and limits. Understanding how to alter workouts ensures that elders may benefit from physical activity while reducing dangers.

- **Adaptations to Improve Joint Health:** To safeguard joint health, low-impact alternatives or sitting forms of activities may be used. Water workouts are very easy on the joints.
- **Creating Your Cardio Workouts:** Adapting cardiovascular workouts to meet endurance levels allows seniors to participate in heart-healthy activities without pushing themselves too far.
- **Strength Training Alterations:** Seniors may gain muscle without risking injury by varying the degree and resistance of strength training activities. Prioritize excellent form above high weights.

## Warm-Up and Cool-Down Routines

The beginning and postlude of any workout regimen are similar to an elegant dance in the field of physical fitness, and they play an important role in maximizing performance, reducing injuries, and boosting general well-being. Warm-up and cool-down exercises are essential components that set the tone for a happy and safe workout session. We dive into the relevance of warm-up and cool-down routines in this research, unraveling their separate functions and providing light on why they are essential to every fitness plan.

- **The Warm-Up:** Getting Your Body Ready for Action A good warm-up is a gradual awakening, a subtle invitation for the body to shift from a state of rest to one of energetic involvement.

- **Improved Blood Flow and Oxygen Delivery:** The warm-up causes an increase in heart rate and blood flow to the muscles. This process ensures that oxygen and necessary nutrients reach the working muscles, preparing them for maximum performance.

- **Joint Flexibility Improvement:** Stretching gently during the warm-up helps to develop joint flexibility. This is especially important for seniors since it helps to offset the natural stiffness that comes with age and increases versatility in motion.

- **Getting the Nervous System to Work:** The warm-up stimulates the neurological system, resulting in a more alert condition. This activation enhances coordination, response speed, and neuromuscular pathway efficiency, resulting in improved overall physical performance.

- **Mental Preparedness:** The warm-up functions as a mental shift in addition to the physical part. It helps people to concentrate on the next activity, creating a conscious connection between the body and future practice.

- **Warm-up Elements that Work Cardiovascular Activity:** Light aerobic exercises like brisk walking, jumping jacks, or cycling progressively raise the heart rate, preparing the cardiovascular system for increasing demands.

- **Stretching Dynamic:** Dynamic stretches that match the motions of the next exercise increase joint flexibility and muscle suppleness.

- **Mobilization in Collaboration:** Gentle joint motions assist in lubricating joints and lessen the chance of tension, especially for regions that will be significantly engaged in the exercise.

- **A Serene Farewell to Intensity:** The cool-down is the tranquil antithesis of the warm-up's energetic overture. It is a purposeful transition from the intensity of exercise to a state of calm, assisting the body in the healing process and decreasing post-exercise discomfort.

- **Heart Rate Gradual Reduction:** The cool-down process comprises a progressive decrease in heart rate, which allows the circulatory system to effortlessly move from a heightened to a more relaxed state.

- **How to Avoid Dizziness and Faintness:** Sudden halts in strenuous physical exercise might cause dizziness or fainting. The cool-down period offers a slow taper down, reducing unpleasant post-exercise symptoms.

- **Improving Metabolic Byproduct Removal:** The body generates metabolic byproducts such as lactic acid during exercise. The cool-down aids in the elimination of these metabolites, lowering the chance of muscular stiffness and pain.

- **Flexibility Maintenance:** Static stretching during the cool-down period helps to maintain and improve flexibility. This may aid in muscle healing and the prevention of long-term stiffness.

# The Following Are the Components of an Effective Cool-Down

1. **Cardio Exercise at a Low Intensity:** Gradually decreasing exercise intensity via low-impact activities assists the body in transitioning to a state of rest.
2. **Stretching at rest:** Static stretches that concentrate on the key muscle groups engaged throughout the exercise help to maintain flexibility and relaxation.
3. **Breathing deeply and being mindful:** Deep breathing exercises and mindfulness practices used during the cool-down help with mental relaxation, stress reduction, and general well-being.

> *In the rhythm of warm-up and cool-down, our bodies find harmony - a prelude to strength and a graceful encore to a workout well done.*

# CHAPTER 2

## NECK AND SHOULDER STRETCHES

## STRETCH #1: NECK FLEXION STRETCH
HOW TO:

- Sit up straight in your chair, shoulders back and down.

- Bring your chin as close to your chest as you feel comfortable. A stretch will be felt at the back of your neck.

- Place your hands on the back of your head and apply slight pressure to improve the stretch.

- Hold for the specified amount of time.

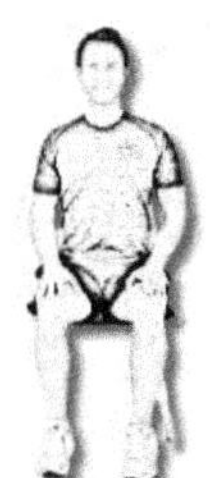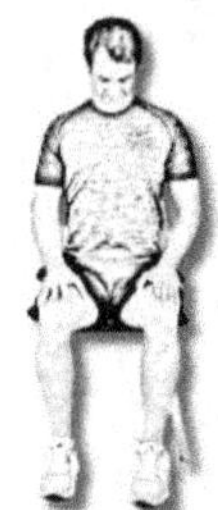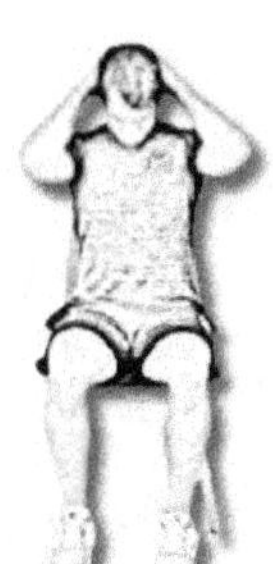

Hold For: 30 Seconds

## STRETCH #2: NECK EXTENSION STRETCH
HOW TO:

- Sit up straight in your chair, shoulders back and down.

- Bring your head back as far as you feel comfortable, staring up at the ceiling. Do not force yourself into discomfort.

- Hold for the specified amount of time.

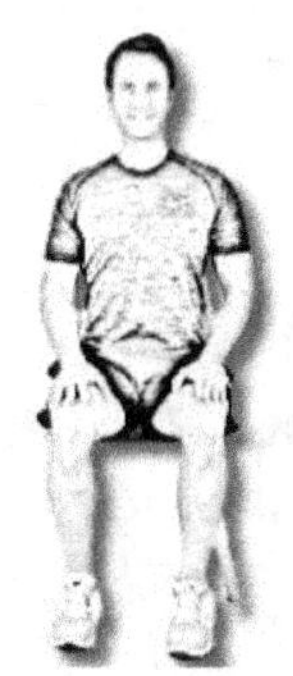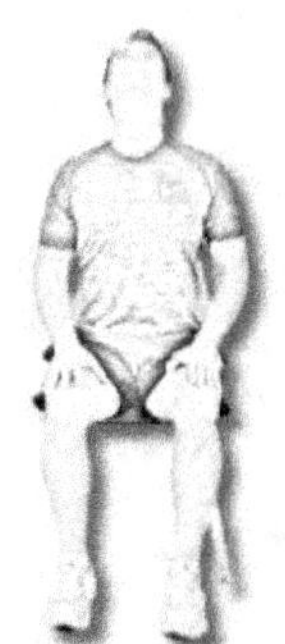

Hold For: 30 - 60 Seconds

# STRETCH #3: NECK SIDE FLEXION STRETCH

## HOW TO:

- Sit up straight in your chair, shoulders back and down.

- Bring your ear all the way down to your shoulder. Do not lift your shoulder up to your ear; instead, keep it relaxed. Go as far as you are comfortable with.

- Place your palm on the side of your head and apply slight pressure to improve the stretch.

- Hold for the specified amount of time, then switch sides.

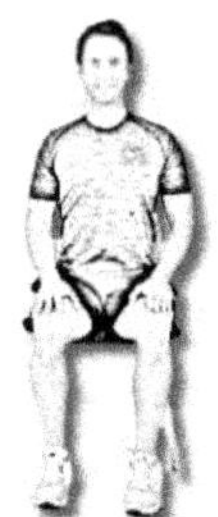 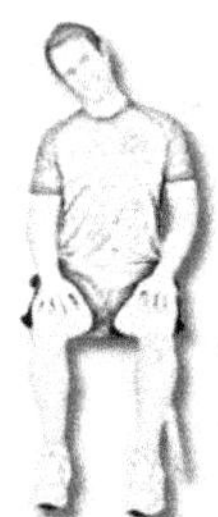 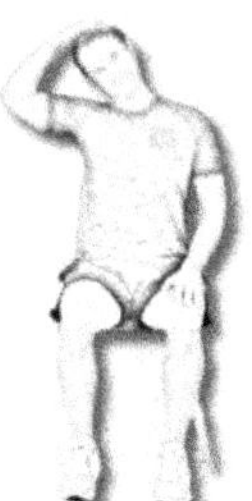

Hold For: 30 - 60 Seconds

# STRETCH #4: NECK ROTATION STRETCH

## HOW TO:

- Sit up straight in your chair, shoulders back and down.

- Look to one side as far as you are comfortable with.

- Hold for the specified amount of time before repeating on the opposing side.

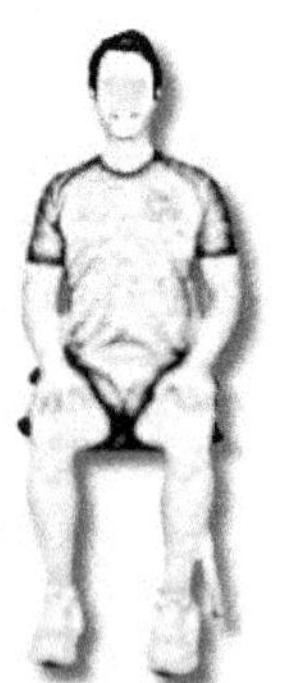 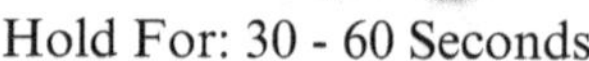 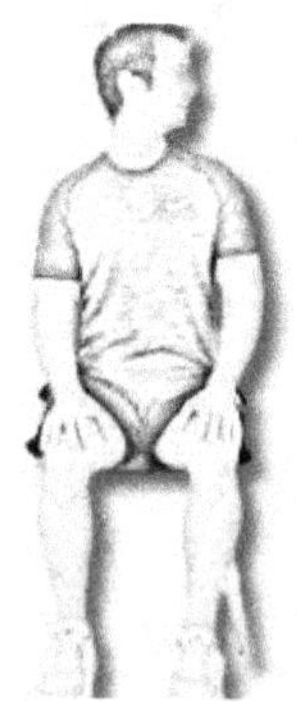

Hold For: 30 - 60 Seconds

# STRETCH #5: LEVATOR SCAPULAR STRETCH

## HOW TO:

- Sit up straight in your chair, shoulders back and down.
- To stabilize your shoulder blade, place the hand on the side you're extending behind it.
- If you are unable to do so, just execute the exercise without one hand behind your shoulder.
- Turn your head 45 degrees to one side and lower your head as if staring at your knee on that side.
- You will feel a stretch behind the neck and shoulder on the opposite side you are looking at. (This is known as the Levator Scapular muscle.)
- Place your palm on the back of your head and apply slight pressure to improve the stretch.
- Hold for the specified amount of time before repeating on the opposing side.

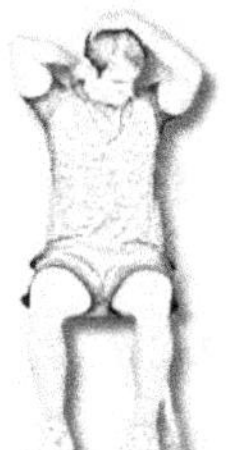

Hold For: 30 - 60 Seconds

## ARM STRETCHES FOR SENIORS

## STRETCH #1: UPPER ARM & SHOULDER STRETCH

## HOW TO:

- Sit tall in your chair, shoulders back and down.
- Place one arm straight in front of your body and use your other hand to embrace the straight arm to your body. This will increase the stretch.
- Hold for the specified amount of time and then switch sides.

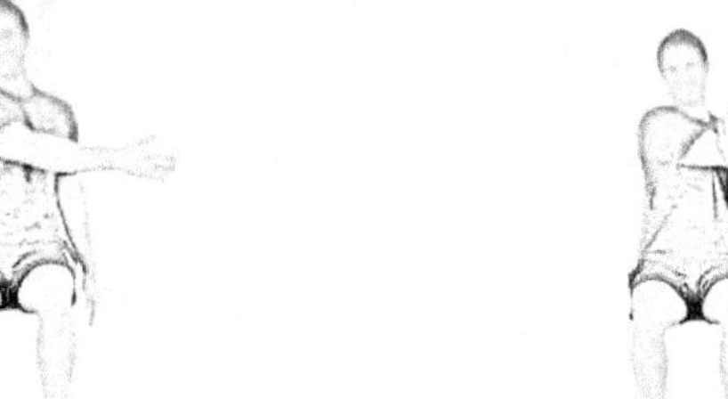

Hold For: 30 - 60 Seconds

## STRETCH #2: SHOULDER & ARM OVERHEAD STRETCH

## HOW TO:

- Sit tall in your chair, shoulders back and down.

- Interlace your fingers and raise your arms over your head.

- Turn your hands away from you, towards the ceiling, and push up as far as you can.

- Hold this action for the designated amount of time, feeling the stretch in your shoulders and sides. sides.

 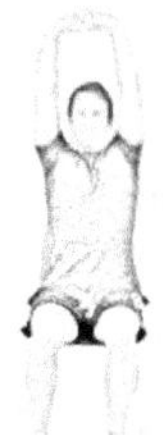

Hold For: 30 - 60 Seconds

## STRETCH #3: WRIST FLEXION (FOREARM) STRETCH

## HOW TO:

- Sit up straight in your chair, shoulders back and down.

- Place one arm straight in front of your body, palm down, and fingers up.

- Drop your wrist, allowing it to weaken.

- Bend your wrist with your other hand, exerting mild pressure on the back of the hand and bringing the hand and fingers towards the elbow. Maintain a straight back during the stretch.

- Hold for the specified amount of time before repeating on the opposing side.

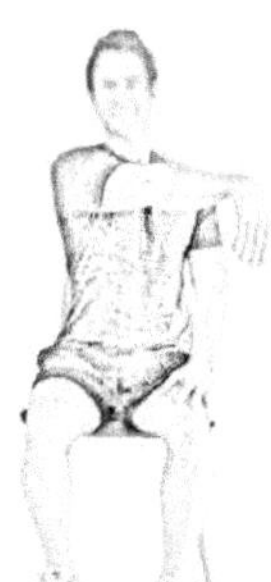 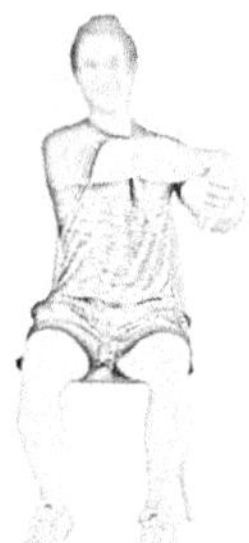

Hold For: 30 - 60 Seconds

# STRETCH #4: WRIST EXTENSION (FOREARM) STRETCH
HOW TO:

- Sit up straight in your chair, shoulders back and down.

- Place one arm straight in front of your body, palm down, and fingers up.

- Bend your wrist with your other hand, providing mild pressure on the fingers towards the elbow. Maintain a straight back during the stretch.

- Hold for the specified amount of time before repeating on the opposing side.

Hold For: 30 - 60 Seconds

# BACK STRETCHES

## STRETCH #1: LUMBAR FLEXION STRETCH (SEATED TOE TOUCH)

HOW TO:

- Sit up straight in your chair, shoulders back and down.

- Place your hands on your knees and your feet slightly out in front of you. Slid your hands down your legs, all the way to your feet, slowly.

- Hold for the specified amount of time, then gently move your hands back up.

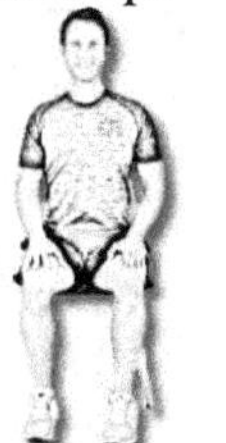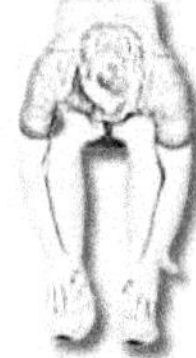

Hold For: 30 - 60 Seconds

# STRETCH #2: LUMBAR SIDE FLEXION STRETCH

## HOW TO:

- Sit up straight in your chair, shoulders back and down.
- Place one hand behind your head and the other just behind you.
- Slowly lower your straight arm until you feel a stretch on the other side.
- (If you have problems putting your hand behind your head, keep it on your lap).
- Hold for the specified amount of time before repeating on the opposing side.

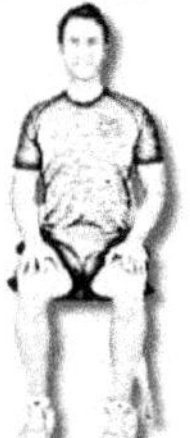 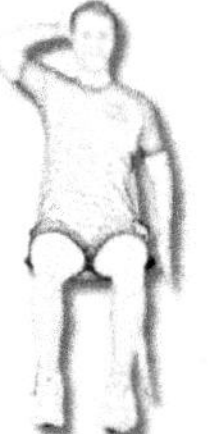 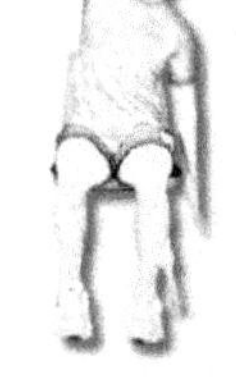

Hold For: 30 - 60 Seconds

# STRETCH #3: LUMBAR EXTENSION STRETCH

## HOW TO:

- Sit up straight in the center of your chair, shoulders back and down.

- Place your palms on the small of your back and lean your lower back into your hands until you feel a stretch in your lower back. (If you have trouble reaching your palms around to the small of your back, use the backs of your hands).

- Hold for the specified amount of time

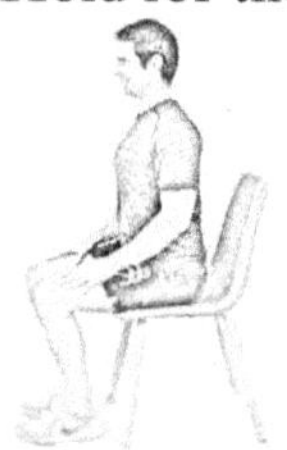 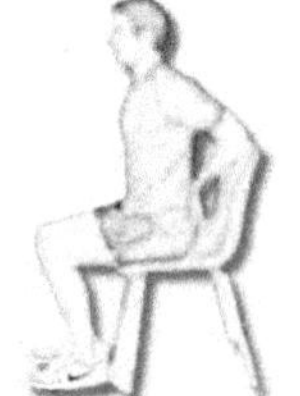 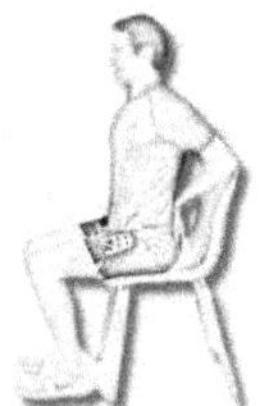

Hold For: 30 - 60 Seconds

# STRETCH #4: RHOMBOIDS (UPPER BACK) STRETCH

HOW TO:

- Sit up straight in your chair, shoulders back and down.

- Put your fingers together and extend your palms away from you.

- Bring your arms up to 90 degrees (or parallel to the floor) and extend your hands as far as possible while remaining upright. Feeling your shoulder blades separate.

- Hold for the specified amount of time before returning to the starting position.

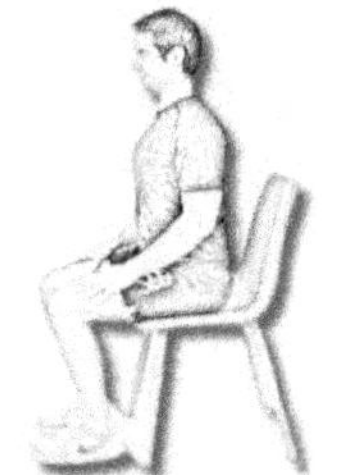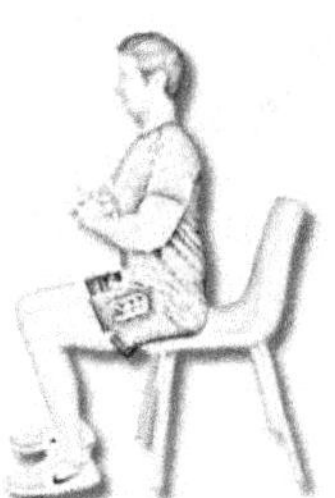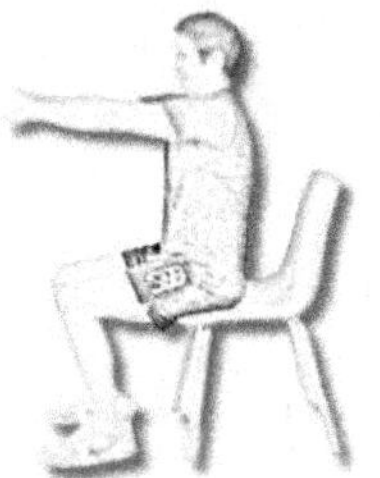

Hold For: 30 - 60 Seconds

# STETCH #5: THORACIC EXTENSION (UPPER BACK)

HOW TO:

- Sit upright in your chair, shoulders back and down.

- Maintain an erect posture and stretch your upper back over the chair by placing your hands behind your head. (If you have problems putting your arms behind your head, place them over your chest).

- Hold for the time specified.

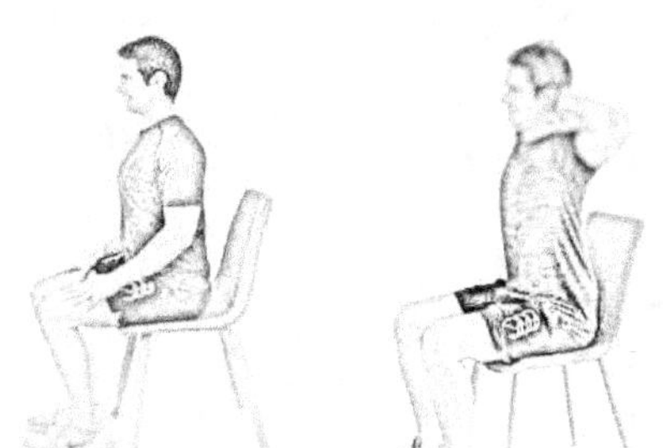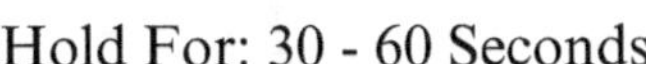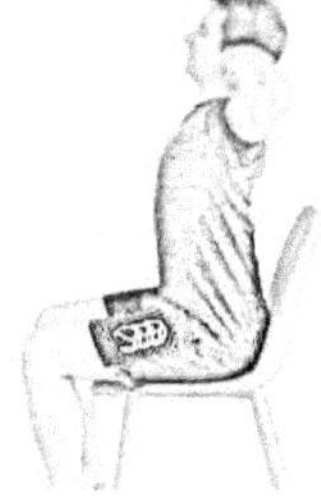

Hold For: 30 - 60 Seconds

# STRETCH #6: THORACIC ROTATION (UPPER BACK)
## HOW TO:

- Sit up straight in your chair, shoulders back and down.

- Cross your arms over your chest and circle around, leading with your arms, until you feel a stretch in your upper back.

- Hold for the specified amount of time before repeating on the opposing side.

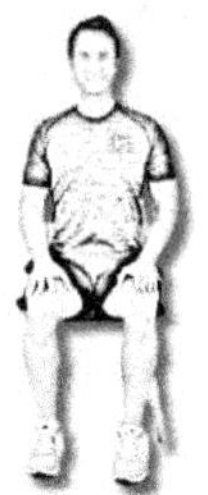 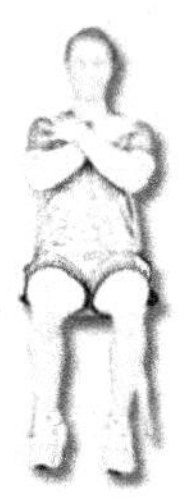 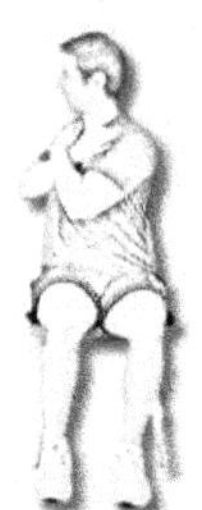

Hold For: 30 - 60 Seconds

# LEG STRETCHE

## STRETCH #1: SEATED HAMSTRING (BACK OF THIGH)
## HOW TO:

- Sit up straight in your chair and shuffle to the front.

- Place one leg out in front of you while keeping your hands on the other leg.

- Maintain a straight leg and point your toes towards the ceiling.

- Maintain a straight spine and bend forward at the hips while remaining upright.

- Hold for the specified amount of time before switching legs.

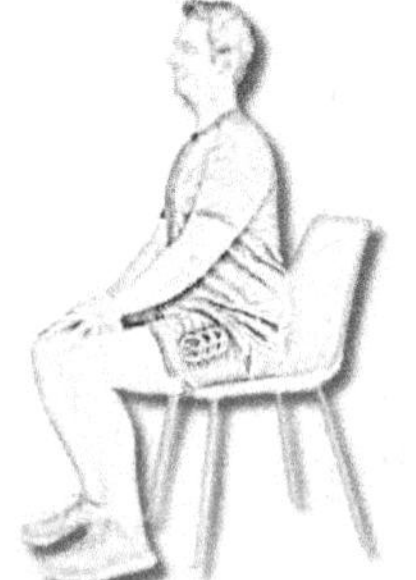 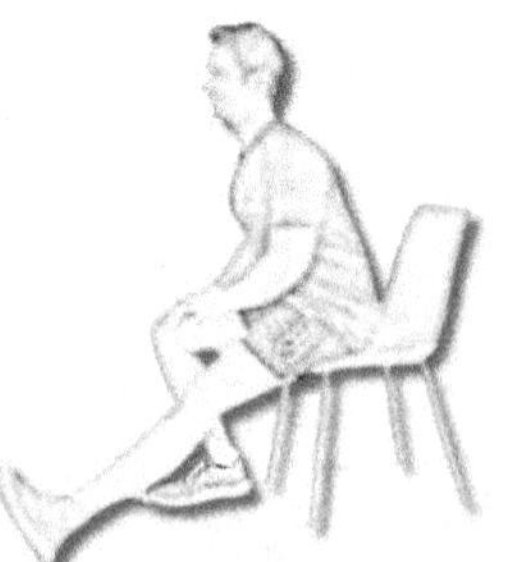 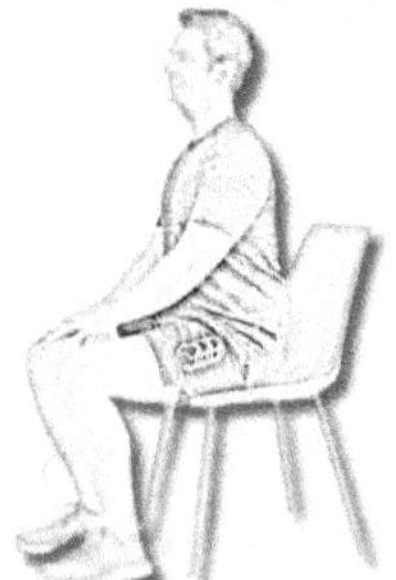

Hold For: 30 - 60 Seconds

# STRETCH #2: SEATED GROIN (HIP ADDUCTOR)

## HOW TO:

- Sit up straight in your chair and shuffle to the front.

- Place one leg out straight to the side, toes on both feet firmly on the ground and looking forward.

- You will feel a stretch on the inner thigh of your straight leg; bend forward slightly to intensify the stretch.

- Maintain an erect posture with a straight back throughout the activity.

- Hold for the specified amount of time before switching legs.

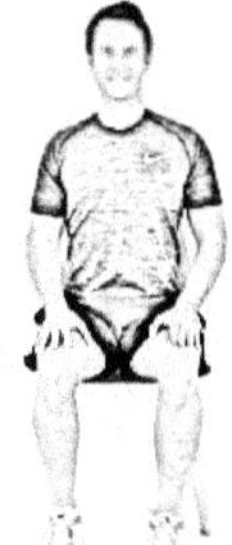 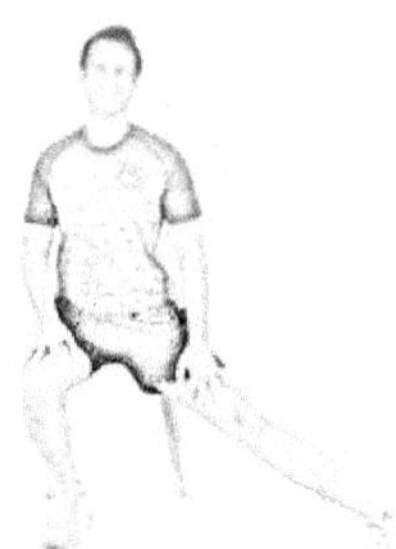

Hold For: 30 - 60 Seconds

# STRETCH #3: SEATED LATERAL ROTATION (HIPS, BUTTOCKS) STRETCH

## HOW TO:

- Sitting up straight, shuffle to the front of your chair.

- Extend your legs and cross one leg over the other while holding onto the chair.

- Slide your heel up your shin until it is in a calm and controlled motion above the kneecap.

- Bend your opposing leg up and place your hands on your shins, keeping your back straight.

- Continue in this posture, and for an extra stretch, lean forward while maintaining your chest up and your shoulders parallel to the floor.

- Hold for the specified amount of time before switching legs.

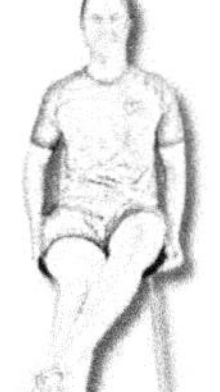 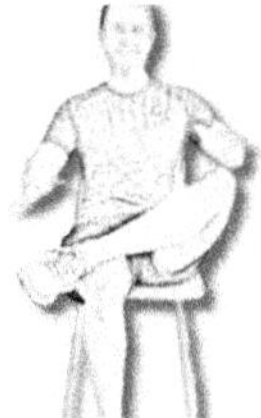 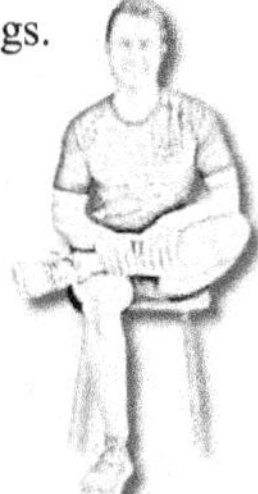

Hold For: 30 - 60 Seconds

# STRETCH #4: HIP FLEXION (BUTTOCKS) STRETCH

## HOW TO:

- Sit up straight, shoulders back and down.

- Hug one leg up to your chest while bending at the knee.

- Hold for the specified amount of time before switching legs.

- Throughout the workout, keep your shoulders back and down.

- Hold for the specified amount of time before switching legs.

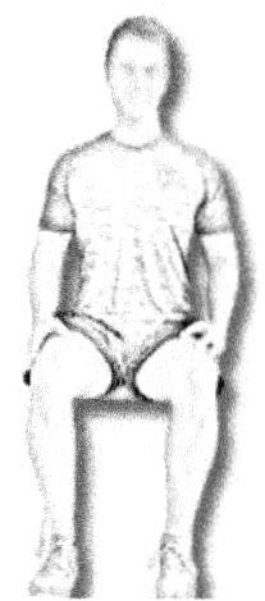 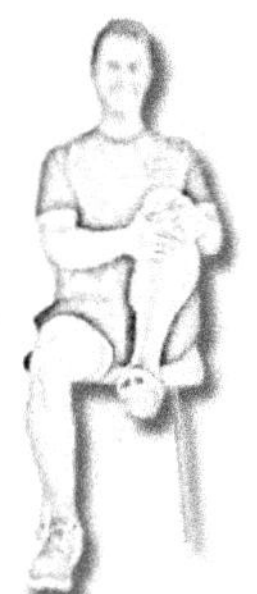

Hold For: 30 - 60 Seconds

# STRETCH #5: STANDING QUADRICEPS (FRONT OF THIGH) STRETCH

## HOW TO:

- Standing tall next to your chair and hanging on with one arm.

- Bring one leg behind you while gripping your foot.

- Maintain a straight posture during the workout and aim to keep your knees close together.

- Hold for the specified amount of time before switching legs.

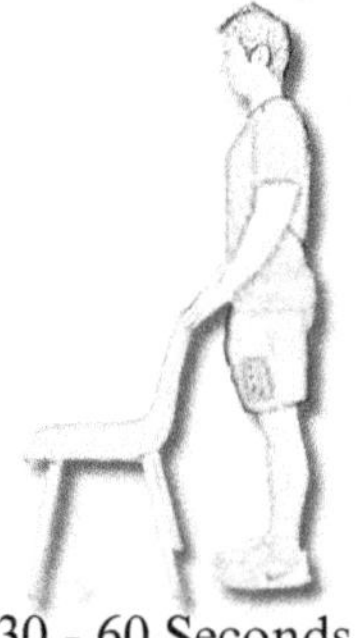 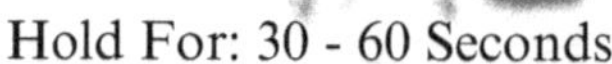 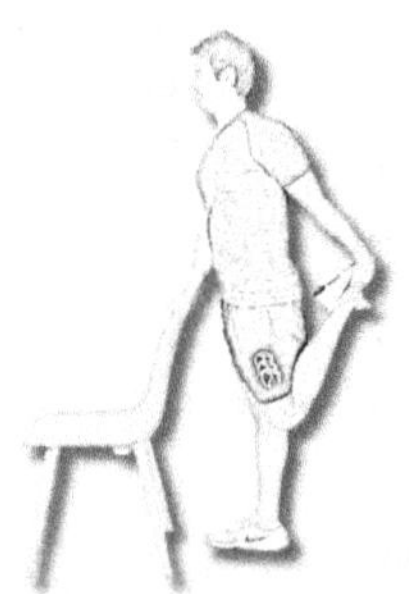

Hold For: 30 - 60 Seconds

# STRETCH #6: STANDING CALF (BACK OF LOWER LEG) STRETCH

HOW TO:
- Standing tall and gripping your chair with both hands.

- Step one foot back, keeping your toes pointed forward throughout the exercise.

- Bring your front knee up to the chair, keeping your heels in touch with the floor at all times.

- Hold for the specified amount of time before switching legs.

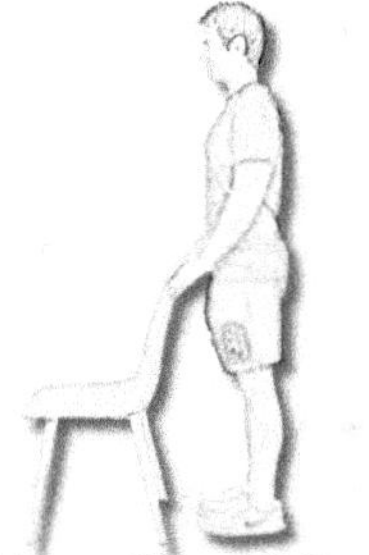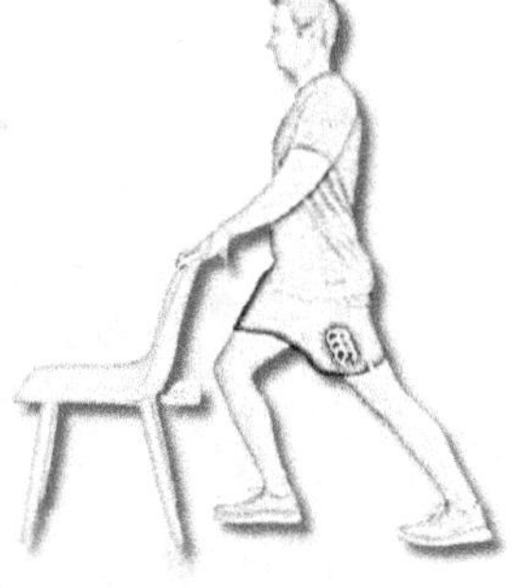

Hold For: 30 - 60 Seconds

Keep in mind that exercise is medicine. It will take a little while to notice a significant increase in your flexibility after you start moving more and incorporate stretching for 10 to 20 minutes every day, or at least three days a week. Everyday mobility will become much simpler for you, and whatever pain you experience will subside. Reaching for objects in those difficult-to-reach areas will be possible. You'll begin to realize just how many advantages come with increased flexibility. You'll experience a return to your former self! Continue to be optimistic as you work toward being a more flexible, active, and healthy version of yourself. Continue to be joyful! And continue to stretch and move! You'll soon get all of your flexibility back and more!

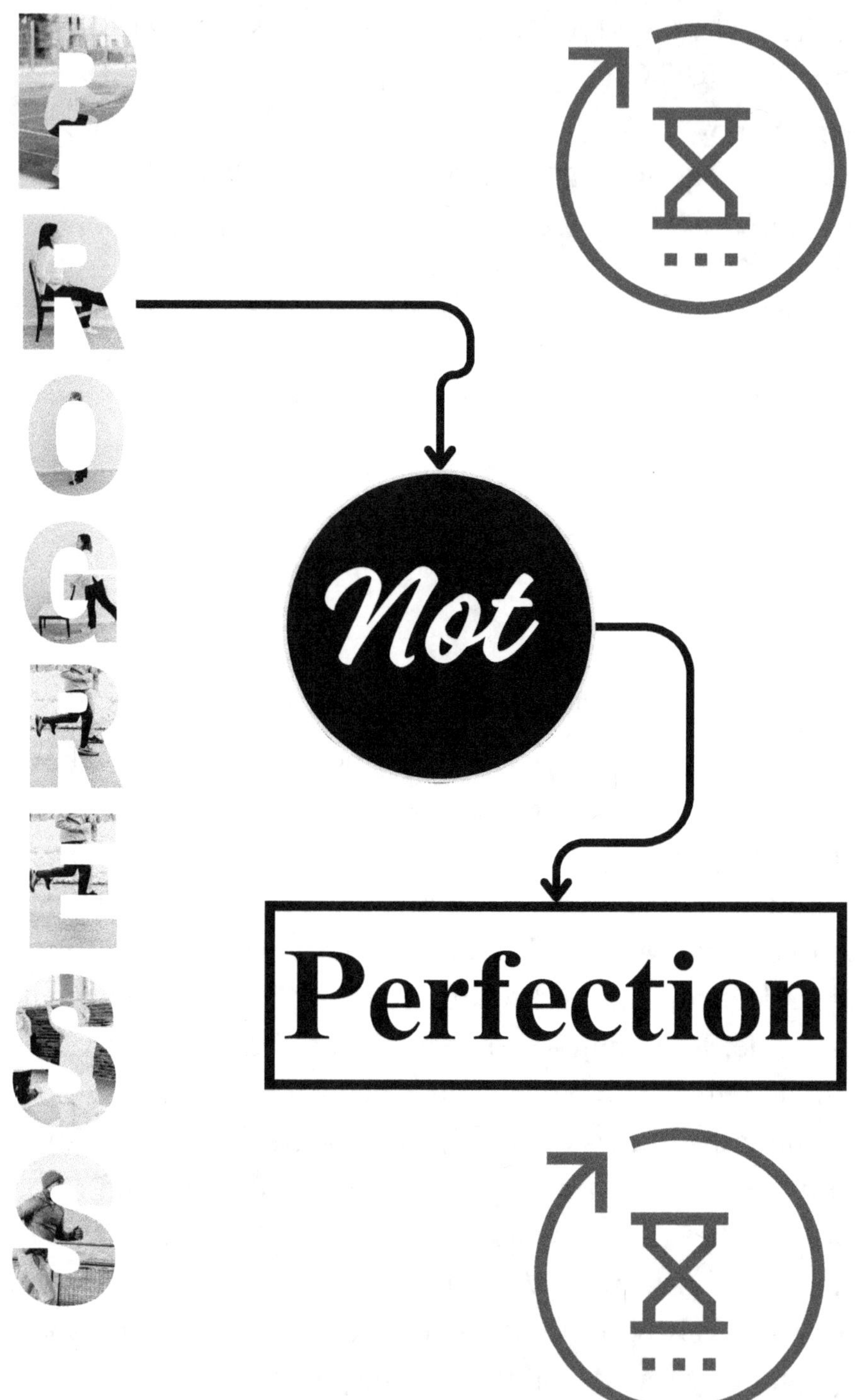

PROGRESS
Not
Perfection

# CHAPTER 3

## BALANCE AND STABILITY EXERCISES

Good balance is vital for staying on your feet, avoiding falls, and making the most of life! You can go through your days with ease if you have an excellent balance! However, as we age, our equilibrium tends to deteriorate, making life more difficult (not to mention deadly)! However, *BALANCE IS A SKILL! A SKILL THAT CAN BE LEARNED AGAIN AT ANY AGE! And, NO MATTER WHAT YOUR CURRENT CAPABILITIES ARE, YOU CAN IMPROVE YOUR BALANCE!*

In this Chapter, you will learn all you need to know to improve your balance, show you how to assess your present balance, and give you everything you need to start balance training and keep you balanced well for life!

All from the convenience of your own home! You don't need any particular equipment or to join a gym. It's simple and may be pleasant. Oh, and by following the exercises in this chapter, you will not only improve your balance, but you will also get stronger, and fitter, look better, feel better, and gain confidence!

We're going to make great strides!

So, let's get balancing!

_Note_ Before we begin, keep in mind that this instruction will only be useful if you use the tactics outlined. Simply reading what's here and performing the exercises once won't help you improve your balance.

Commit to add at least 5-10 minutes of balancing practice into your weekly routine. Make things as easy as possible. Make it enjoyable!

**WHY DOES BALANCE CHANGED AS WE AGE?**

We must realize that certain circumstances are beyond our control. That is, changes in our bodies (physiological changes) occur due to aging. We will never return to our 20- or 30-year-old selves again.

The good news is that the fundamental contribution to these physiological changes is not aging itself, but rather that we do less as we age. As we enter adulthood, the strains of life begin to take grip, and we find ourselves with additional responsibilities.

We also develop bad habits (for example, sitting in bad postures more frequently), and we engage in less and less physical exercise. Many of us attribute the physical changes we see (such as diminished balance, posture, and strength, among other things) to aging. However, the majority of the time, these changes occur due to reduced exercise over time.

We witness many of these changes in our physical state simply because we sit more and walk less.

We are creatures of comfort, created to do what is most comfortable, and doing more exercise gets harder with time.

**Physical changes caused by inactivity include:**

- Weakness all throughout the body.
- A general loss of fitness (our whole body becomes less fit, resulting in quicker muscular exhaustion and shortness of breath).
- Change our center of mass by lowering our stance.
- Balance has been compromised.

It's time to admit that the major reason keeping active and upright has gotten more difficult and you're not moving as well as you could isn't because of aging, but because we've done less and less movement over time.

You must remove the notion that impaired balance and falls are typical aspects of aging from your mind. This is a mythology.

*FALLS CAN BE PREVENTED AND YOUR BALANCE CAN BE IMPROVED.*

Now that we know this, we should do all we can to enhance our balance and maintain it that way in the future for the numerous advantages it will offer us.

# HOW TO CHECK YOUR BALANCE

There are several tests that may be used to assess balance.

The goal of assessing your balance is to gain a basic idea of how well you can balance and then use these measurements to track your development after conducting balance training.

I picked four tests to give you a general idea of your balance.

However, before we begin the testing, you will require the following fundamental equipment:

**YOU WILL NEED THE FOLLOWING EQUIPMENT:**

To adequately evaluate and develop your balance, I suggest the following:

- A measuring tape
- Timer This means that you may use your mobile phone as a timer.
- Chair - A standard chair with arms. It's not a sofa.
- A strong piece of furniture (e.g., kitchen bench, rail, etc.).
- A helper - enlist the assistance of a family member, friend, or workout partner to assist with the measurements.
- A Wall.

# BALANCE EXAMINATION

Let's get started with the testing.

**<u>TEST #1 - BALANCE TEST WITH FOUR POINTS</u>**

A timer and a chair are required for the test.

***Test Specifications*:**

This first test is a static balance test (balance when stationary). This test will put your balance to the test in four progressively challenging foot positions.

***How to Carry Out the Test:***

- For safety concerns, stand close to the back of a chair, a rail, or a substantial piece of furniture (e.g., a kitchen bench).
- Begin by gripping the chair and assuming the first foot position of the test (see below).
- When you're ready, remove your hands from the chair and begin the timer. Perform this test without clinging to the chair.

- Throughout the test, you may move your arms to maintain balance (holding onto the surface if necessary). The test is halted when your feet move out of place, and the time is recorded in the chart below.

- If you can safely hold the position for 30 seconds, go on to the next tough foot position, and so on until you reach the last (4th) foot position.
- For single-foot stances, alternate feet.
- Record your findings in the table that follows this section

***PLEASE NOTE:*** If you are unable to complete the test in 30 seconds for this foot position, stop the test and note your time.

If you are unable to sustain 30 seconds for foot positions 1 and 2, continue to practice and train these actions until you can safely handle 30 seconds for each before proceeding.

If you are not improving, see your doctor or a physiotherapist for a more tailored regimen.

Find the joy of resilience in every stretch." Quick exercises with many options.

## FOOT POSITION 1) The feet Side-by-side:

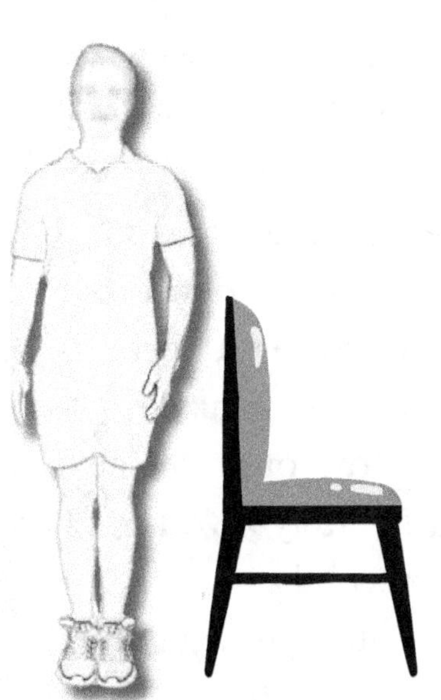

- Feet as near together and side by side as feasible.
- For safety reasons, have a chair or rail near by.
- Hold for at least 30 seconds, or as long as you can.
- If you can maintain the position for 30 seconds, you may safely advance to the next position.

## FOOT POSITION #2) SEMI TANDEM STANCE

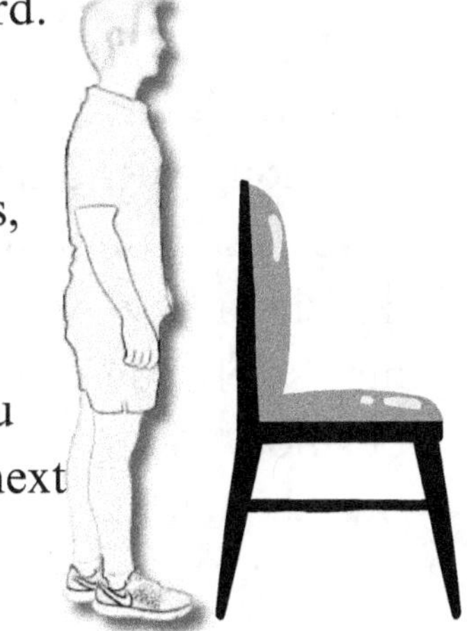

- Stand placing one foot's big toe in the arch of the other.
- The toes are pointed forward.
- For safety reasons, have a chair or rail nearby.
- Hold for at least 30 seconds, or as long as you can.
- If you can maintain the position for 30 seconds, you may safely advance to the next position.
- Switch your feet.

## FOOT STAND #3) TANDEM STANCE

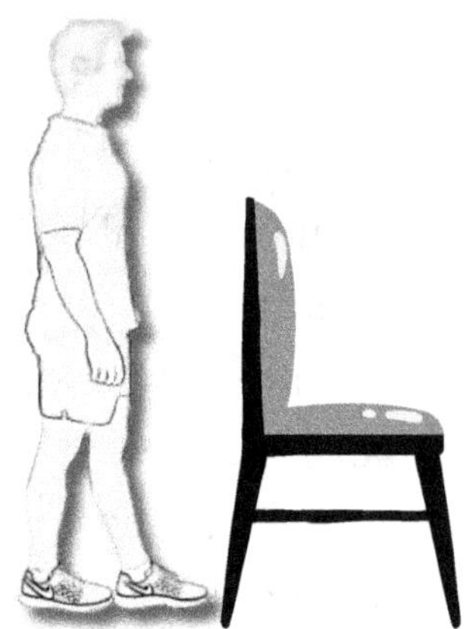

- Standing upright with one foot's heel touching the toes of the other.
- For safety reasons, have a chair or rail nearby.
- Hold for 30 seconds, or for as long as you can.
- Move on to the next position securely if you can hold for 30 seconds.
- Alternate your feet.

## FOOT POSITION #4) SINGLE LEGGED STANCE

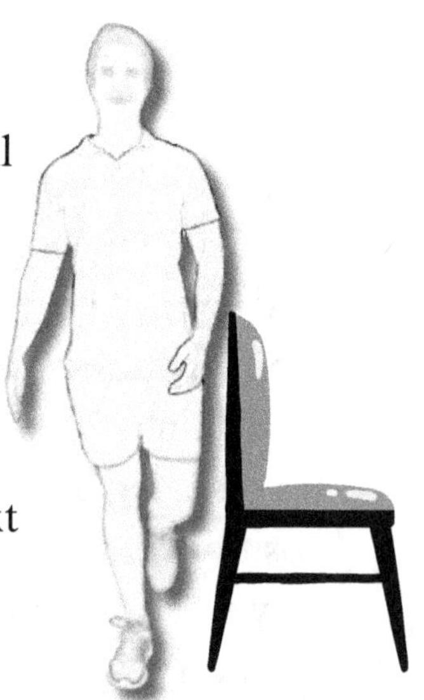

- The one leg Standing.
- For safety, have a chair or rail nearby.
- Hold for at least 30 seconds, or as long as you can.
- If you can maintain the position for 30 seconds, you may safely advance to the next position.
- Switch your feet.

# Evaluating Your Results

A score of 30 seconds on each test indicates that your balance is adequate for the given test.

You can always improve, no matter what your strengths are. To do this, you must increase the difficulty of the balancing training (described later).

There is always work to be done.

If you score fewer than 30 seconds on any of the tests, don't be too harsh on yourself; it just shows you need to practice your balance more.

Don't worry if you score lower on one side than the other (for example, your left foot versus your right foot); this is normal.

You are more likely to tumble if you are over 60 and score fewer than 10 seconds on the tandem stand.

Whatever your outcomes are, write them down with the intention of improving them following your training time.

> **Embrace the energy inside. Quick exercises are your daily dose of elder strength.**

<u>**TEST #2 - STANDING REACH**</u>

***Equipment Needed:***

A chair, a bare wall, a tape measure, and a helper are all required for safety.

Before you begin, keep in mind that you may use a tape measure to help you.

***<u>Test Specifics:</u>***

The standing reach test is intended to examine our balance when standing and reaching for things.

**How to Carry Out the Test:**

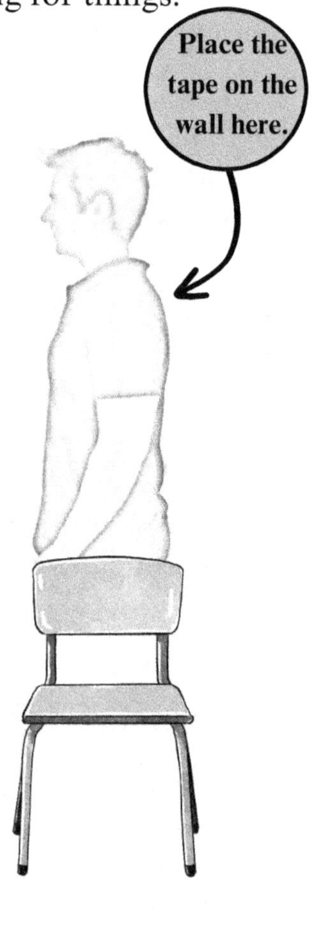


- Place a piece of tape on the wall at the level of your shoulder while standing perpendicular to it. This is a reference to your starting point.
- For your own protection, have a chair nearby.
- Now, stand perpendicular to the piece of tape and about 15 cm from the wall, with your feet hip-width apart and staring straight ahead.
- Lift your arm to 90 degrees, parallel to the floor, using the arm closest to the wall. Keep your hand in a fist and remain comfortable, with neither your feet nor your body shifting out of place.

- With a piece of tape, mark the location of your knuckle on the wall. This is the starting position (Y).

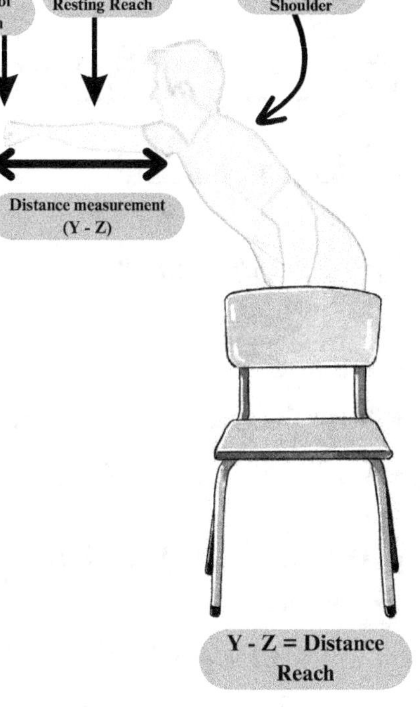


- Reach out in front of you as far as you can while maintaining your arms parallel to the floor.
- Maintain your equilibrium by not allowing your feet to move out of place. Position Z is the ultimate reach position.
- Once you've reached as far as you can, have the person assisting you mark the knuckle of your fist with a piece of tape.
- Make careful you don't overextend yourself and lose your equilibrium.
- View in full-size
- Balance testing using a reach test Y - Z = Reach Distance
- Using the tape measure, measure the distance between the two tape locations and note the findings in the table below.

- Complete a practice run before taking the exam three times.
- Calculate the average of the three tests and save the findings for further use.

# TEST #3 - TIMED UP AND GO

***Equipment Needed***

A chair, a tape measure, tape, and a helper.

***Test Specifications***:

The Time Up and Go puts our balance and mobility to the test once again.

You will stand from a chair, move 3 meters over a line, turn around, go back to the chair, and sit.

## How to Carry out the Test:

- Make sure you have a friend or family member to assist you with this exam.
- A buddy can take a more exact assessment of the time it takes you to complete the test, and it's also a good idea to have someone present for safety concerns if your balance isn't so excellent.
- As with any balancing tests, make sure they don't help you with any aspects of the exam, but having someone standing beside you is a good idea.
- Position your chair in an open area of your home that is level and free of impediments or trip risks.

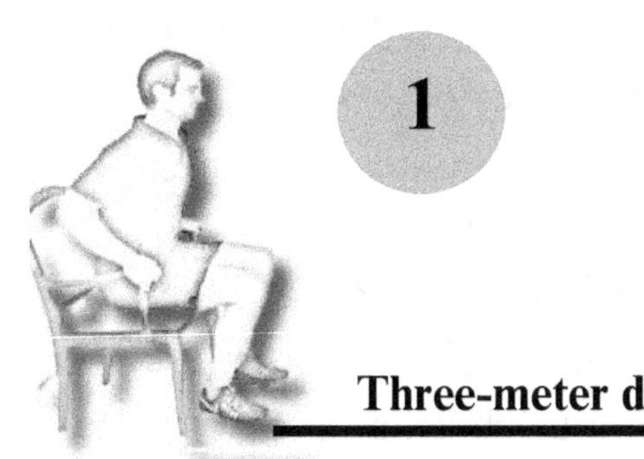

1
Three-meter distance


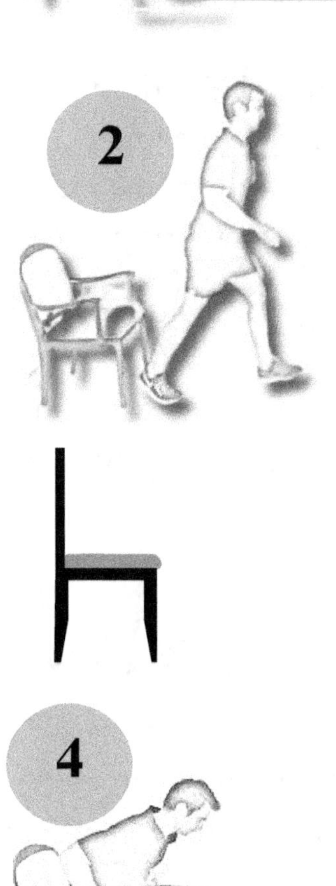

2
4


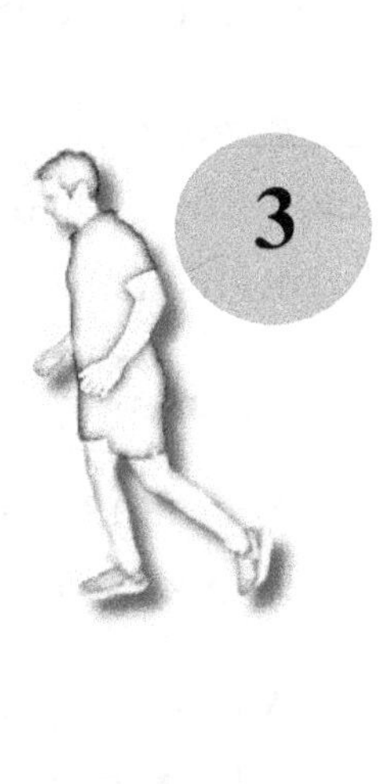

3

- Using your tape measure, mark 3 meters from the chair and mark it with a piece of tape.
- Sit in the chair with your hands on the armrests and your back against the backrest.
- Your assistant will yell "GO" and start the timer. You must get out of your chair, go to the line, turn around, walk back to your chair, and then sit again. Walk at your regular speed.
- When your buttocks contact the chair, the test is complete, and your assistant will stop the timer.
- Perform a practice run of the exam to get the feel of it, but allow enough time before the scoring test to ensure you are not exhausted.
- Run this test twice and average the results

***Take note***: If you normally use walking assistance (such as a walking stick or walker), utilize it throughout the test.

**Understanding Your Outcomes:**

- According to research, if your time is longer than 13.5 seconds, you are more likely to fall

- Whatever your outcomes are, write them down with the goal of improving them with balancing training

# TEST #4 - Sit to Stand For Five Minutes

***Equipment Needed***

Chair, Timer, and a helper.

***Test Specifications***:

This test measures the power and strength of our lower limbs. It's a functional examination because we spend much of our day sitting and standing in chairs.

The duration of this test is the amount of time it takes you to stand and sit five times.

## How to Carry Out the Test:

- Allow someone to time you, or hold the timer in your hand.
- Begin by sitting in the chair.
- You will time how long it takes you to rise up and sit down. [The test (and the timer) will begin as soon as your buttocks leave the chair. And when your buttocks are on the chair after the fifth stand, stop the timer (complete the test).
- Cross your arms over your chest without gripping the armrests. The feet should be hip-width apart. [It's all right if you need to grab the armrests. Take notice of it, however. You will most likely discover that after exercising and strengthening your balance and strength, you will no longer need to hang on.]
- When standing, make sure your knees and hips are straight and that the back of your knees are not contacting the chair.

- Sit down calmly, rather than collapsing down into the chair.
- Practice one stand and one sit before beginning the five tries to get the idea of the test but don't overdo it.
- Carry out this exam and note all findings for future reference.

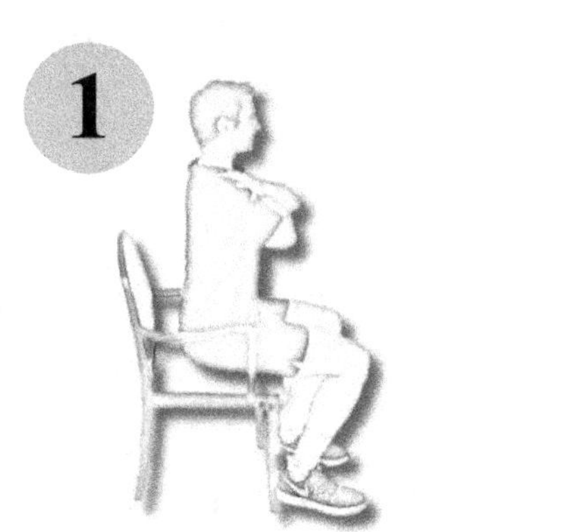
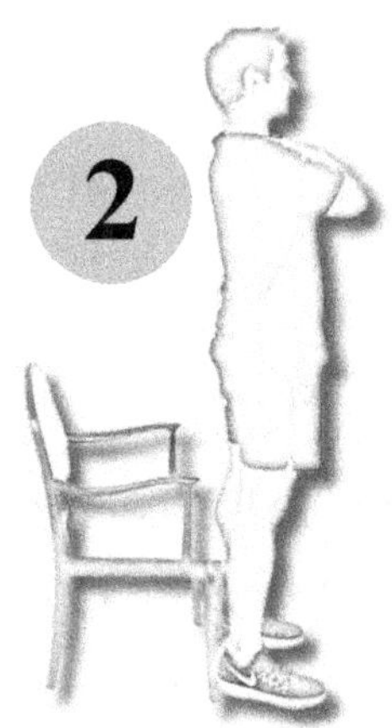

**Understanding Your Outcomes**

The following are the standard age range measurements
- 60 to 69 years old: 11.4 seconds.
- 70 to 79 years old: 12.6 seconds.
- The testing process takes 14.8 seconds for those aged 80 to 89.

Regardless of your outcomes, even if you are unable to execute one sit-to-stand. Write it down to improve it once you've trained your balance.

# CHAPTER 4

## STRENGTH TRAINING FOR SENIORS

Strength training may benefit everyone, but it is particularly good for seniors. Building and maintaining body strength helps to keep your bones healthy, increases mobility and stability, avoids falls, and relieves arthritic pain. It may also be a pleasant and satisfying method to keep active. With these advantages in mind, we've compiled a list of five strength training exercises for seniors that you may do at home.

Before beginning a new workout plan, consult with your doctor or a fitness professional to ensure appropriate technique.

1. ***Body weight Exercises***

- **SQUATS**

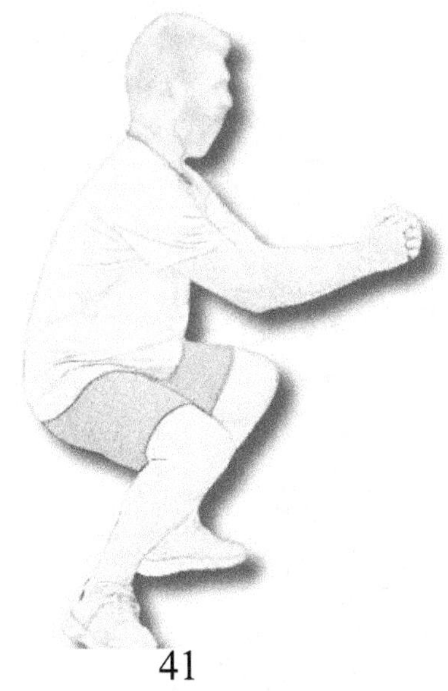

Squatting helps to develop your whole lower body and core, making actions like climbing stairs and lifting items up off the floor simpler and safer. To begin this exercise, stand straight in front of a firm chair. Place your feet slightly wider than shoulder-width apart and your arms parallel to the ground. As you count to five, gently bend your knees and lower yourself towards the chair, taking care not to stretch your knees past your toes. While the chair is there to catch you if you fall, avoid sitting and instead hover above the seat. Pause. Then, as you count to three, gently return to a standing posture. Repeat.

- **WALL PUSH UP'S**

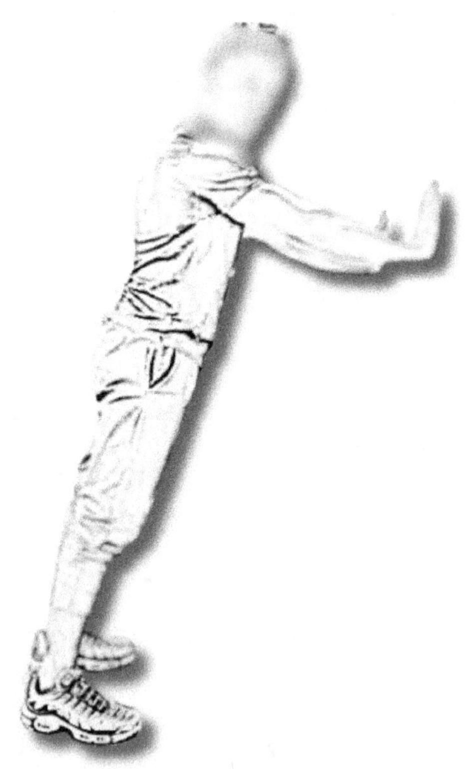

This senior strength training exercise is a modified version of the basic floor push-ups you may remember from physical education class as a child. Find a blank wall and stand at least an arm's length away. Lean forward and rest your hands flat on the wall at approximately shoulder-length and shoulder-width apart, facing the wall. Bend your elbows as you drop your upper body softly toward the wall. Count to five while keeping your feet firmly in place. Pause, then gently push yourself back until your arms are straight once again. You can do these wall push-ups up to ten times, or as many as you find difficult.

- **DEAD BUGS**

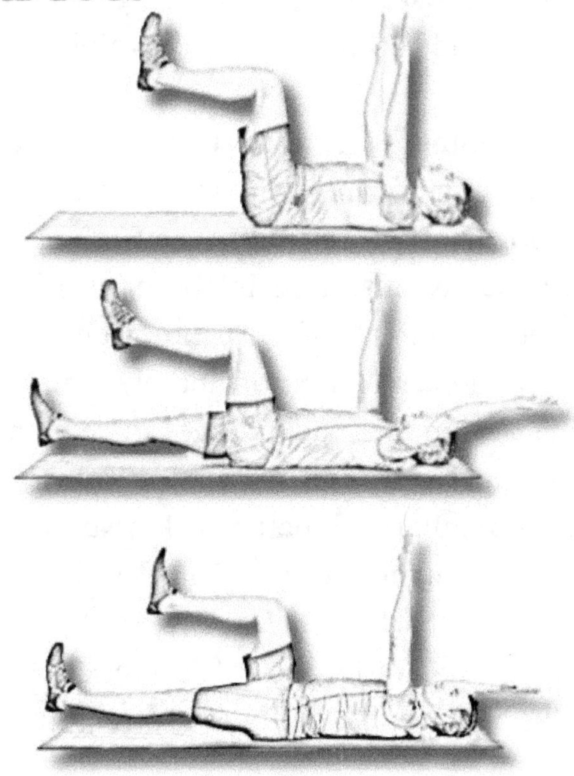

To do a dead bug exercise, lay flat on your back with your arms and legs up in the air, knees bent. Press the small of your back against the floor. Lower one leg toward the floor and the opposing arm behind you, maintaining your core strong and knees bent. Pause, then return to the starting point. Repeat with the opposite arm and leg as many times as your body permits without discomfort or strain.

### *2. Light Resistance Band Excercise*

Resistance training, often known as strength training, is a kind of exercise that improves physical strength and endurance. Muscles are pushed to move against tension produced by body weight, dumbbells, gravity, machines, or resistance bands during resistance training.

Resistance training, when included in a regular exercise regimen, may significantly enhance muscular strength, balance, coordination, flexibility, and range of motion. Resistance exercise also aids in the prevention of bone loss and the symptoms of arthritic discomfort. senior-resistance-band-exercisesUnfortunately, many seniors are missing out on these advantages since many persons over the age of 70 do not exercise at all. Even people who exercise regularly sometimes skip strength training in favor of walking or another sort of cardio.

However, the greatest kind of exercise is a mix of aerobic plus balance, flexibility, and strength training.

Resistance workouts are still useful for seniors. In fact, the American College of Sports Medicine and the American Heart Association recommend that seniors (65 and over) exercise for at least 150 minutes per week, or 2 and a half hours per week, and involve weight training at least twice a week. There are several resources available to help you get started with resistance training. Resistance bands are ideal for seniors since they are lightweight, simple to transport, and inexpensive.

Resistance bands are strong, elastic bands that may be used to train all of the body's muscles. Some resistance bands feature grips on the ends, whereas others do not. They also come in a variety of resistance levels according to your degree of fitness. Choose the one that works best for you and gradually raise the tension of the resistance band as your fitness level improves.

Resistance bands may be used to do a variety of strength workouts, including chest presses, rows, shoulder presses, bicep curls, and tricep extensions. The advantages of employing resistance bands are many.

**Here are just a handful of the advantages of using resistance bands in your training program**

- Resistance bands are inexpensive.
- Resistance bands are often cheap, frequently costing less than $10. For less than $50, some resistance bands contain DVDs, additional fitness equipment, and a guidebook.

- Resistance bands are appropriate for people of varying fitness levels. Resistance bands may be used by anybody, young or old, novice or expert. The intensity level is easily adjustable with a range of resistances: low, medium, and heavy.
- Resistance bands work out the whole body. Every major muscle group is worked by resistance bands. As a result, they may be utilized for total-body training.
- Resistance bands are simple to keep. The bands take up very little space, making them simple to use and store even in small spaces.
- Resistance bands may be used to offer diversity. To give muscles a respite, resistance bands may be alternated with lightweight dumbbells or training equipment.
- Resistance bands may be utilized at any time and in any place. They are lightweight and compact, allowing them to be transported anywhere.
- Resistance bands are an efficient exercise tool.
- Resistance bands are a basic idea, yet they are incredibly effective for boosting strength and endurance, as well as stamina, flexibility, and balance.

# BICEP CURLES

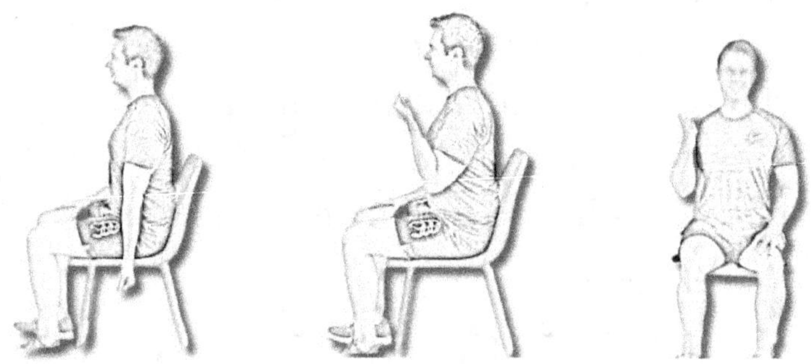

- Curl your arm from the elbow all the way up to the top and then gently drop it back down.
- Rep the given number of times, switching arms.

- Make sure your arm is completely straightened on the way down and fully bent on the way up.
- This exercise may also be performed with both arms simultaneously.

THE MUSCLES WORKED
- Biceps (forearms), Forearms, and Deltoids (shoulders)

# SEATED ROWS

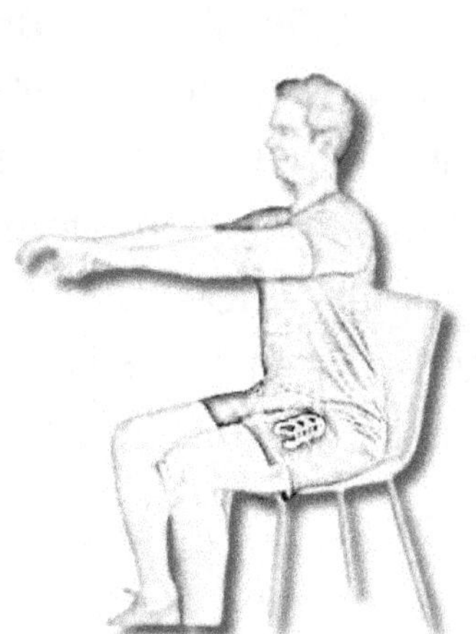
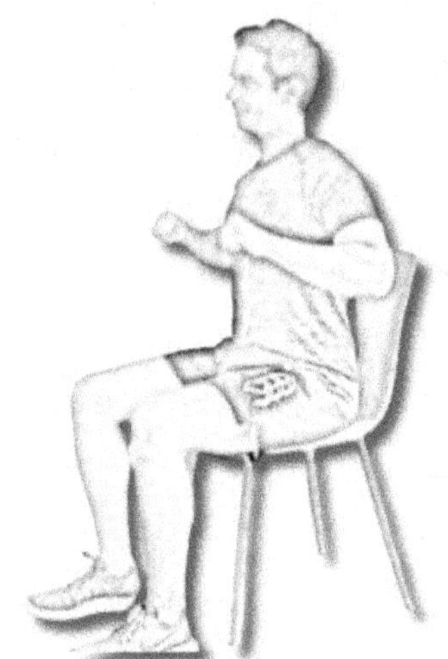

- Sit up straight in your chair.
- Spread your arms in front of you.
- Pull your elbows behind you, pressing your shoulder blades together at the finish. remember to keep your chest up the whole time.
- repeat for the specified number of times.

THE MUSCLES WORKED

- Arms, shoulders, and the back.

## Selecting the Right Resistance Level

You should be aware of your strength and fitness level before purchasing resistance cables. Begin with your present fitness level, not the fitness level you wish to achieve.  Select a resistance that you can utilize without departing from the appropriate form. You don't want to damage yourself by changing your body mechanics, nor do you want to grow disheartened because the workout is too difficult.

Extra-light resistance cables are advised for the elderly or those recovering from an injury or sickness. Light resistance cables are ideal for rehab, elderly ladies, and teenagers who are just beginning their exercise adventure. Medium resistance cords are an excellent spot to begin resuming a fitness plan or daily training. Heavy cords can be used by active men and women who are practicing for their particular sports.

# CHAPTER 5

**Mindfulness and Relaxation Techniques**

Maintaining your health and fitness is essential at any age, especially as you become older. If you want to decrease stress, reflect, or alleviate health concerns like high blood pressure or sleeplessness, mindfulness could be for you.

Mindfulness is the discipline of paying attention to your thoughts, feelings, and experiences, which encompasses many different mental exercises and meditations. Mindfulness stresses living in the present moment and cultivating inner tranquility. You may be completely aware of yourself and the environment around you if you take the time to ponder, relax, and focus.

## HOW CAN SENIORS BENEFIT FROM MINDFULNESS?

Mindfulness offers several advantages that can improve one's health and well-being. If you make mindfulness a practice in your life, you may notice some of the following advantages:

- Enhanced emotional well-being
- Increased inner peace
- Anxiety and despair have been reduced.
- Lower blood pressure in hypertensive patients
- Less mood swings
- Better eating and exercise habits
- Improved sleep quality and fewer symptoms of insomnia
- Improved quality of life when dealing with chronic disease

**Senior Mindfulness Exercise And Meditation**

Mindful Breathing: Sit, stand, or sleep comfortably, preferably with your eyes closed, and bring awareness to your breath as you inhale and exhale. Take note of how your body feels as you breathe in and then out. If your mind wanders, bring it back to the breath. Begin with a few minutes and work your way up to five to seven minutes every day.

- **Mindful Body Awareness:** While sitting or resting comfortably, bring your attention to your body and all of its components, beginning with your feet and working your way up. Notice any feelings, thoughts, or emotions you may be experiencing, and release any tension in your body. Choose a calm and deserted location or trail and begin walking gently. Keep your concentration on the feeling of walking and how you feel as you take steps and maintain balance. Be in the moment and enjoy wandering without a destination.
- **Mindful Movement:** Exercises such as tai chi, sitting chair stretches, and yoga promote the mind-body connection while easing stress. Incorporate your breathing methods and pay attention to how your body feels while executing each activity.
- **Mindful Eating:** Begin with a small amount of food, such as a raisin or a bit of chocolate, and focus on how it looks, feels, and smells. Once you've put it in your mouth, pay close attention to the texture and flavor. Make a conscious effort to eat slowly, relish every bite, and be appreciative of the meal you're consuming.

- **Mindful Guided Meditation:** Those new to the practice may benefit from adopting a guided meditation. Here are some of our favorite mindfulness apps: Headspace, Aura, Buddhify, Calm, or Insight Timer are all options.

According to studies, these workouts can create major changes in the brain after only eight weeks of constant practice. These changes include an increase in gray brain matter associated with memory; a thickening of the left hippocampus, which aids in learning, cognition, and emotional regulation; and a decrease in the size of the amygdala, the "fight or flight" part of the brain, which correlates to a reduction in stress levels. We recommend giving mindfulness a try and encourage your loved ones to do the same!

## Incorporating Mindfulness Into Our Daily Life

These are easy techniques for incorporating mindfulness into your daily life, but they are not the only ones. If you're seeking for other solutions, consider yoga, deep breathing exercises, a gratitude practice, and ways to connect with your inner child and engage in play. Remember that finding the mindfulness techniques that work best for you or resonate the most with you may take some time and experimentation.

Speaking with a therapist is another approach to learn more about mindfulness. Many people have heard of mindfulness exercises for dealing with stress, anxiety, and other difficulties.

Some even employ mindfulness-based stress reduction treatment and other methods that include mindfulness practices. According to research, this treatment that integrates these approaches can help people enhance their degree of mindfulness and even reduce symptoms of anxiety and depression—even when done online.

If you're interested in this type of online treatment, you may look for it on a site like BetterHelp.

**Here are some basic yet effective ways to incorporate mindfulness into your everyday routine:**

**Mindful Breathing:** Start each day with some mindful breathing. Take a seat, close your eyes, and concentrate on your breathing. Slowly inhale, feeling the air enter your body, and expel with intention. This mindful breathing sets a pleasant tone for the rest of the day.

**Daily Reflection:** Set aside some time each evening to reflect on the events of the day. Recognize and express thankfulness for minor pleasures, and analyze obstacles carefully and without judgment. This introspective exercise promotes mindfulness and emotional equilibrium.

**Thoughtful Walking:** Turn a simple stroll into a thoughtful exercise, whether indoors or outdoors. Feel the experience of each step, pay attention to your body's small motions, and engage your senses in the surroundings around you.

Walking attentively helps you connect with the present moment and relax.

**Mealtime Ritual**: Make mealtime a thoughtful ritual. Appreciate the colors, textures, and scents of your cuisine to engage your senses. Chew gently and thoroughly. This method not only improves meal satisfaction but also supports good digestion.

**Guided Meditation**: Work brief guided meditations into your daily practice. Many online platforms provide guided lessons tailored exclusively for elders. These workshops offer moderate direction for relaxation, stress reduction, and mindfulness cultivation.

**Nature Connection:** Spend time in nature and be immersed in its splendor. Nature provides a quiet backdrop for mindful reflection, whether it's a stroll in the park, sitting in a garden, or listening to the sounds of birds.

**Mindful Stretching or Yoga:** Practice moderate stretching or yoga movements while paying attention to each movement and sensation in your body. This exercise and mindfulness combo improves flexibility, balance, and overall well-being.

These easy techniques integrate mindfulness into routines, generating a sense of calm and improving general quality of life.

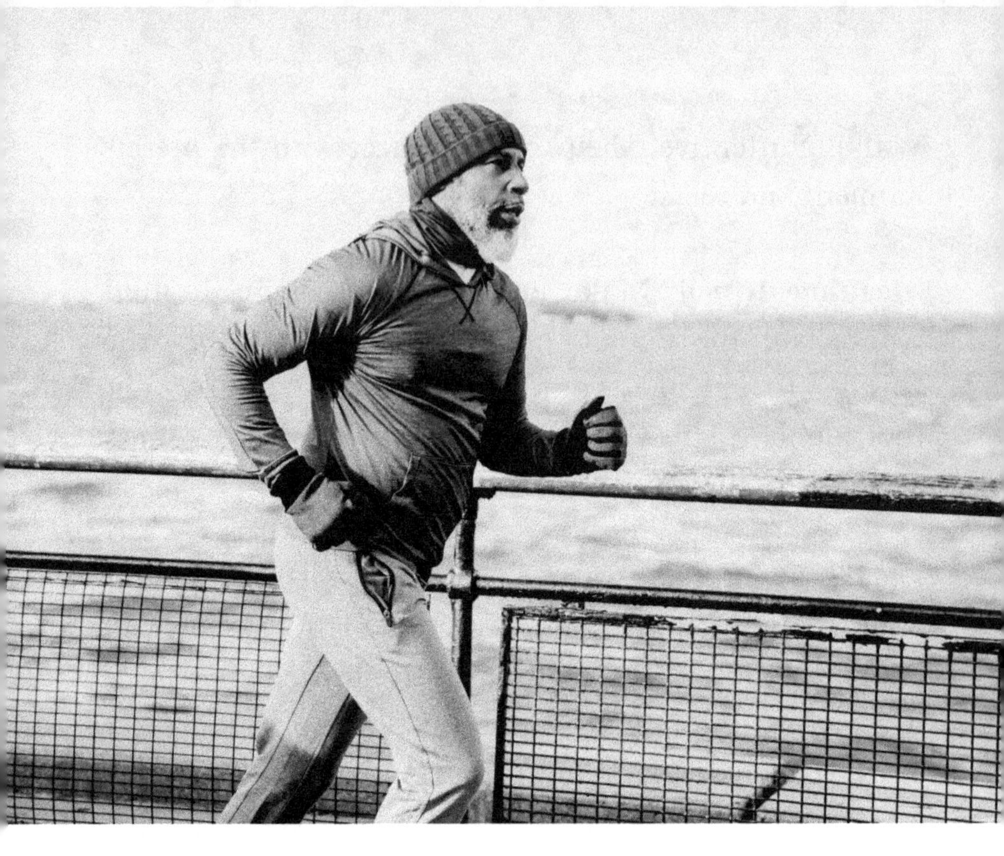

**"Even if it's only for a short while, make it a point to engage in some form of physical activity each day. You'll be more inclined to follow your regimen in this way."**

# CHAPTER 6

## Creating a Sustainable Routine

Developing a long-term fitness program for seniors is a deliberate effort that promotes long-term well-being. It entails a planned combination of exercises, individual needs attention, and a commitment to regularity. A consistent regimen recognizes seniors' particular health profiles and develops a good engagement with exercise.

First, an assessment of individual requirements and health circumstances is required. Consultation with healthcare specialists ensures that the routine is adapted to individual issues and objectives. A well-rounded approach is ensured by the incorporation of a range of exercises, such as cardiovascular activities, strength training, and flexibility exercises.

Starting gently and gradually is critical for avoiding injuries and increasing adherence. A steady schedule, whether daily or many times per week, is the foundation of a long-term habit. Flexibility is essential for allowing for changes as needs change throughout time.
Enjoyable activities add to the routine's long-term viability. Choosing activities that provide delight, whether it's dancing, strolling, or group workouts, guarantees that seniors are more likely to continue with their program.

Social involvement, such as participating in group classes or exercising with friends, adds a motivating factor and promotes a feeling of community

Prioritizing rest and recuperation days, rewarding accomplishments, and including regular health check-ins ensure that the program is in line with personal health goals.

## Setting Realistic Fitness Goals in a Senior Workout

Setting Realistic Fitness Goals in a Senior Workout

Setting realistic fitness objectives is an important part of a short workout regimen for seniors since it ensures that expectations match individual capabilities and desired achievements. Realistic goals provide a foundation for growth, motivation, and a sense of success.

First and foremost, goals must be explicit and suited to individual requirements. Specificity aids in the design of focused workouts, whether the goal is to improve cardiovascular health, increase flexibility, or build strength. Seniors can measure progress more successfully when bigger goals are broken down into smaller, attainable milestones.

Realistic goals take into account the timeframe in which they may be achieved. Seniors should be aware of their present fitness level and establish objectives that are hard but achievable in a fair amount of time. Gradual growth is essential for avoiding discouragement and keeping enthusiasm high.

**Establishing a Regular Exercise Schedule**

A consistent exercise program is essential for success in a short workout regimen for seniors. Consistency not only increases the benefits of exercise, but it also fosters a long-term and habitual approach to physical activity.

To begin, while deciding the optimal time for exercise, elders should examine their own preferences and energy levels. Choosing a time that fits with individual habits and seems doable, whether in the morning, afternoon, or evening, provides more adherence.

Making a weekly program with particular days and hours for exercise provides organization. This timetable should be reasonable and adaptable, allowing for other obligations while prioritizing physical exercise. Consistency promotes habit-building, making exercise a part of everyday life.

Including variation in the workout routine reduces boredom and offers a well-rounded approach to fitness. Changing between aerobic, weight training, and flexibility routines not only delivers a balanced workout but also keeps the program new and engaging.

Setting reminders or incorporating exercise into current habits, such as going for a walk after meals, might help with consistency. Having a dedicated gym room, whether at home or in a communal setting, also helps to an easy-to-follow regimen.

Establishing a regular workout plan benefits not only physical health but also mental discipline. Seniors should embrace their exercise program with zeal, understanding that each session adds to their overall health. Regular exercise develops a habit over time, encouraging a healthy and sustainable lifestyle.

**Tracking Progress and Making Adjustments**

Tracking progress and making required modifications are critical components of a short workout regimen for seniors for retaining motivation, guaranteeing continuing growth, and avoiding plateaus. A proactive approach to accomplishment tracking gives useful information into the effectiveness of the workout regimen.

To begin, seniors should develop a method for recording important variables linked to their fitness objectives. This might involve keeping track of the length and intensity of exercises, the number of steps completed, or the amount of weight lifted. Keeping a basic notebook or using fitness apps will help you keep track of your progress.

Regular evaluations of physical qualities such as flexibility, endurance, and strength provide objective measures of progress. Seniors can return to baseline examinations regularly to compare them to their present abilities, offering real evidence of their hard work and devotion.

It is critical to incorporate regular health check-ins with healthcare providers. These check-ins allow for a thorough review of general health, addressing any emergent issues, and ensuring that the fitness program is appropriate for the individual.

When development slows or some workouts become less effective, changes to the regimen are required. Modifying workouts, increasing intensity, or introducing new activities to push the body in new ways might be part of this. The capacity to alter the program guarantees that it stays active and produces great effects.

It's critical to be tuned in to your body's cues. Seniors should pay attention to how their bodies react to exercise, noting any discomfort or changes in their physical well-being. Individual comfort levels can then be accommodated, and overexertion avoided.

When measuring progress and making changes, flexibility and willingness to change are critical mindsets. Seniors should consider these changes as opportunities for growth and refinement rather than setbacks. Finally, a fast workout regimen that changes depending on progress tracking is effective, enjoyable, and suited to individual requirements.

## Staying Motivated for the Long Term

Staying motivated over time is a major issue in any fitness quest, especially for seniors who follow a short training plan. Sustaining motivation necessitates a combination of inner and external variables, as well as a positive mentality that understands the long-term advantages of regular exercise.

Setting realistic and attainable objectives is critical to retaining motivation. Seniors should set goals that are both difficult and attainable, giving them a sense of success as they advance. Celebrating these accomplishments boosts motivation and promotes a good attitude toward exercise.

Workout regimen variety is vital for avoiding boredom and monotony. Seniors can try a variety of exercises, such as water aerobics, yoga, or dance. This provides excitement while simultaneously targeting different muscle areas and increasing overall fitness.

Participating in social fitness activities, such as group classes or exercising with friends, gives a support system. A sense of community and shared goals boosts motivation and responsibility. Having a workout buddy may make training more fun and help you commit to regular sessions.

Reassessing and changing the training regimen regularly helps to avoid plateaus and assures continual improvement. The routine's dynamic nature keeps seniors interested and motivated to take on new tasks. Long-term sustainability requires flexibility in modifying the routine to individual demands.

Including incentives and positive reinforcement is a potent motivator. When seniors reach fitness goals, they may treat themselves to tiny prizes, developing a positive link with exercise. These incentives might be as simple as eating a favorite healthy snack or doing something soothing.

Developing a good mentality is possibly the most important part of long-term motivation. Exercise should be viewed by seniors as a comprehensive investment in their well-being, with physical, mental, and emotional advantages. This viewpoint underlines the long-term importance of a regular fitness regimen, which contributes to a long-term commitment to health and vitality.

> *Every gentle move in your quick workout is a step towards timeless strength*

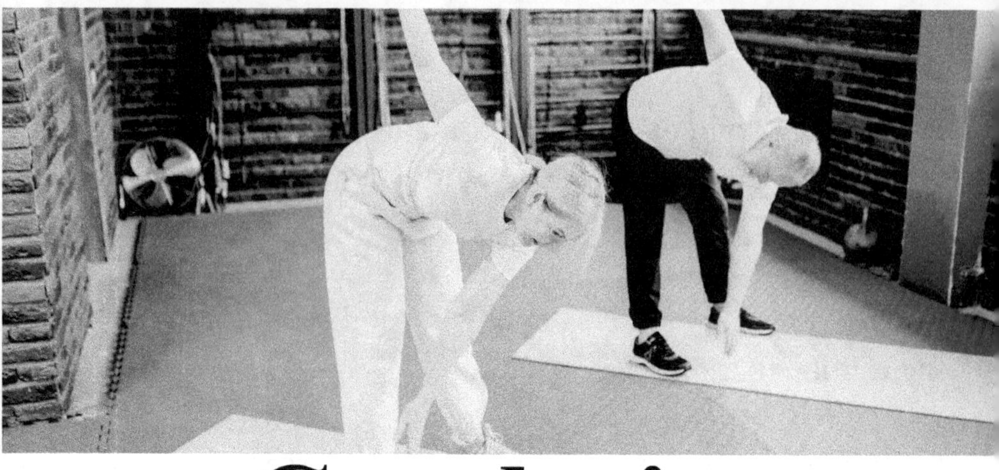

# Conclusion

Begin your adventure to redefine aging with "Quick Workout for Seniors Aged 60+." Say yes to strength, energy, and a future in which you are in control of your health. Your golden years are designed to shine, and this book will help you get there.

Take advantage of the chance immediately. **Click "Add to Cart"** to invest in your health, opening the door to a new chapter of vitality and resilience. Join the thousands of others who have embraced this game-changing approach to senior fitness.

Your feedback is invaluable. Please share your opinions with us after witnessing the beneficial improvements. Your candid feedback not only helps us progress but also motivates other seniors to begin their fitness journey. Let us redefine aging together and celebrate the power of a healthier, happier self.

*Cheers to a prosperous future!*

# TRACK YOUR PROGRESS

Date:_____________________________

| | EXERCISE | GOAL |
|---|---|---|
| **MON DAY** | | |
| **TUES DAY** | | |
| **WEDNES DAY** | | |
| **THURS DAY** | | |
| **FRI DAY** | | |

*Progress Not Perfection!*

# TRACK YOUR PROGRESS

Date:_____________________

| | EXERCISE | GOAL |
|---|---|---|
| **MON DAY** | | |
| **TUES DAY** | | |
| **WEDNES DAY** | | |
| **THURS DAY** | | |
| **FRI DAY** | | |

*Progress Not Perfection!*

# TRACK YOUR PROGRESS

Date:________________________

| | EXERCISE | GOAL |
|---|---|---|
| **MONDAY** | | |
| **TUESDAY** | | |
| **WEDNESDAY** | | |
| **THURSDAY** | | |
| **FRIDAY** | | |

*Progress Not Perfection!*

# TRACK YOUR PROGRESS

Date:_____________________________

| | EXERCISE | GOAL |
|---|---|---|
| **MON DAY** | | |
| **TUES DAY** | | |
| **WEDNES DAY** | | |
| **THURS DAY** | | |
| **FRI DAY** | | |

*Progress Not Perfection!*

# TRACK YOUR PROGRESS

Date:_____________________

| | EXERCISE | GOAL |
|---|---|---|
| **MON DAY** | | |
| **TUES DAY** | | |
| **WEDNES DAY** | | |
| **THURS DAY** | | |
| **FRI DAY** | | |

*Progress Not Perfection!*

# TRACK YOUR PROGRESS

Date:_______________________

| | EXERCISE | GOAL |
|---|---|---|
| **MON DAY** | | |
| **TUES DAY** | | |
| **WEDNES DAY** | | |
| **THURS DAY** | | |
| **FRI DAY** | | |

*Progress Not Perfection!*

# TRACK YOUR PROGRESS

Date:_____________________

| | EXERCISE | GOAL |
|---|---|---|
| **MON DAY** | | |
| **TUES DAY** | | |
| **WEDNES DAY** | | |
| **THURS DAY** | | |
| **FRI DAY** | | |

# TRACK YOUR PROGRESS

Date:_______________________

| | EXERCISE | GOAL |
|---|---|---|
| **MON DAY** | | |
| **TUES DAY** | | |
| **WEDNES DAY** | | |
| **THURS DAY** | | |
| **FRI DAY** | | |

*Progress Not Perfection!*

# TRACK YOUR PROGRESS

Date:______________________

| | EXERCISE | GOAL |
|---|---|---|
| **MON DAY** | | |
| **TUES DAY** | | |
| **WEDNES DAY** | | |
| **THURS DAY** | | |
| **FRI DAY** | | |

*Progress Not Perfection!*

# TRACK YOUR PROGRESS

Date:_____________________

| | EXERCISE | GOAL |
|---|---|---|
| **MON DAY** | | |
| **TUES DAY** | | |
| **WEDNES DAY** | | |
| **THURS DAY** | | |
| **FRI DAY** | | |

*Progress Not Perfection!*

# TRACK YOUR PROGRESS

Date:_____________________________

| | EXERCISE | GOAL |
|---|---|---|
| **MON DAY** | | |
| **TUES DAY** | | |
| **WEDNES DAY** | | |
| **THURS DAY** | | |
| **FRI DAY** | | |

*Progress Not Perfection!*

# TRACK YOUR PROGRESS

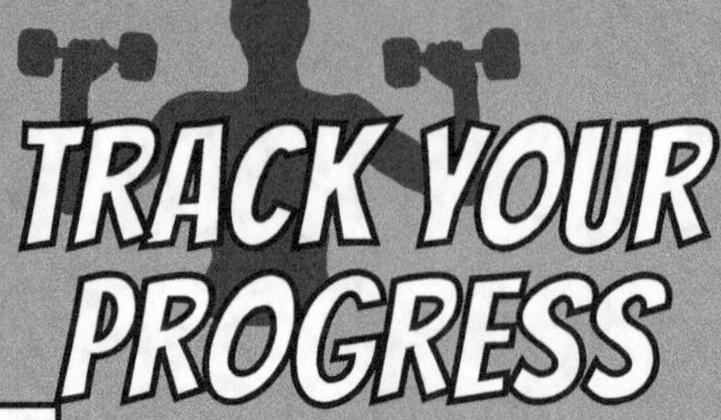

Date:_____________________

|  | EXERCISE | GOAL |
|---|---|---|
| **MONDAY** |  |  |
| **TUESDAY** |  |  |
| **WEDNESDAY** |  |  |
| **THURSDAY** |  |  |
| **FRIDAY** |  |  |

*Progress Not Perfection!*

# TRACK YOUR PROGRESS

Date:_______________________

| | EXERCISE | GOAL |
|---|---|---|
| **MON DAY** | | |
| **TUES DAY** | | |
| **WEDNES DAY** | | |
| **THURS DAY** | | |
| **FRI DAY** | | |

*Progress Not Perfection!*

# TRACK YOUR PROGRESS

Date:_________________________

| | EXERCISE | GOAL |
|---|---|---|
| **MON DAY** | | |
| **TUES DAY** | | |
| **WEDNES DAY** | | |
| **THURS DAY** | | |
| **FRI DAY** | | |

*Progress Not Perfection!*

# TRACK YOUR PROGRESS

Date:_________________________

| | EXERCISE | GOAL |
|---|---|---|
| **MON DAY** | | |
| **TUES DAY** | | |
| **WEDNES DAY** | | |
| **THURS DAY** | | |
| **FRI DAY** | | |

*Progress Not Perfection!*

# TRACK YOUR PROGRESS

Date:_______________________________

| | EXERCISE | GOAL |
|---|---|---|
| **MON DAY** | | |
| **TUES DAY** | | |
| **WEDNES DAY** | | |
| **THURS DAY** | | |
| **FRI DAY** | | |

*Progress Not Perfection!*

# TRACK YOUR PROGRESS

Date:_____________________

| | EXERCISE | GOAL |
|---|---|---|
| **MON DAY** | | |
| **TUES DAY** | | |
| **WEDNES DAY** | | |
| **THURS DAY** | | |
| **FRI DAY** | | |

*Progress Not Perfection!*

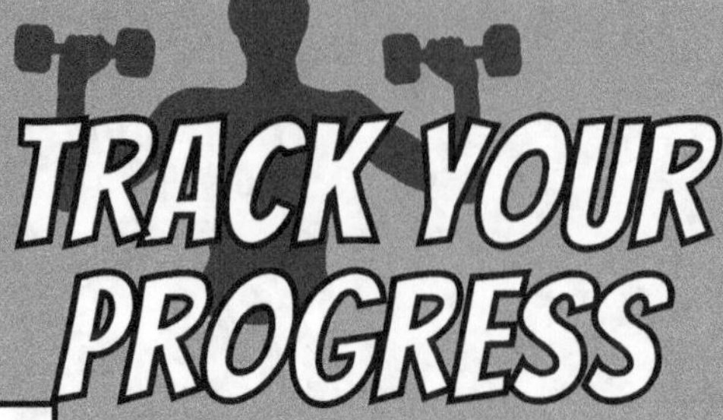


Date:______________________

| | EXERCISE | GOAL |
|---|---|---|
| **MON DAY** | | |
| **TUES DAY** | | |
| **WEDNES DAY** | | |
| **THURS DAY** | | |
| **FRI DAY** | | |

*Progress Not Perfection!*

# TRACK YOUR PROGRESS

Date:_______________________

| | EXERCISE | GOAL |
|---|---|---|
| **MON DAY** | | |
| **TUES DAY** | | |
| **WEDNES DAY** | | |
| **THURS DAY** | | |
| **FRI DAY** | | |

*Progress Not Perfection!*

# TRACK YOUR PROGRESS

Date:_____________________________

| | EXERCISE | GOAL |
|---|---|---|
| **MON DAY** | | |
| **TUES DAY** | | |
| **WEDNES DAY** | | |
| **THURS DAY** | | |
| **FRI DAY** | | |

*Progress Not Perfection!*

# TRACK YOUR PROGRESS

Date:_____________________

| | EXERCISE | GOAL |
|---|---|---|
| **MONDAY** | | |
| **TUESDAY** | | |
| **WEDNESDAY** | | |
| **THURSDAY** | | |
| **FRIDAY** | | |

*Progress Not Perfection!*

# TRACK YOUR PROGRESS

Date:_______________________

|  | EXERCISE | GOAL |
|---|---|---|
| **MON DAY** | | |
| **TUES DAY** | | |
| **WEDNES DAY** | | |
| **THURS DAY** | | |
| **FRI DAY** | | |

*Progress Not Perfection!*

# TRACK YOUR PROGRESS

*Date:*______________________

| | EXERCISE | GOAL |
|---|---|---|
| **MON DAY** | | |
| **TUES DAY** | | |
| **WEDNES DAY** | | |
| **THURS DAY** | | |
| **FRI DAY** | | |

*Progress Not Perfection!*

# TRACK YOUR PROGRESS

Date:_________________________

| | EXERCISE | GOAL |
|---|---|---|
| **MON DAY** | | |
| **TUES DAY** | | |
| **WEDNES DAY** | | |
| **THURS DAY** | | |
| **FRI DAY** | | |

# TRACK YOUR PROGRESS

Date:_______________________

| | EXERCISE | GOAL |
|---|---|---|
| **MON DAY** | | |
| **TUES DAY** | | |
| **WEDNES DAY** | | |
| **THURS DAY** | | |
| **FRI DAY** | | |

*Progress Not Perfection!*

# TRACK YOUR PROGRESS

Date:_____________________

| | EXERCISE | GOAL |
|---|---|---|
| **MON DAY** | | |
| **TUES DAY** | | |
| **WEDNES DAY** | | |
| **THURS DAY** | | |
| **FRI DAY** | | |

*Progress Not Perfection!*

# TRACK YOUR PROGRESS

Date:______________________________

| | EXERCISE | GOAL |
|---|---|---|
| **MON DAY** | | |
| **TUES DAY** | | |
| **WEDNES DAY** | | |
| **THURS DAY** | | |
| **FRI DAY** | | |

*Progress Not Perfection!*

# TRACK YOUR PROGRESS

Date:_____________________

| | EXERCISE | GOAL |
|---|---|---|
| **MON DAY** | | |
| **TUES DAY** | | |
| **WEDNES DAY** | | |
| **THURS DAY** | | |
| **FRI DAY** | | |

*Progress Not Perfection!*

# TRACK YOUR PROGRESS

Date:_________________________

| | EXERCISE | GOAL |
| --- | --- | --- |
| **MON DAY** | | |
| **TUES DAY** | | |
| **WEDNES DAY** | | |
| **THURS DAY** | | |
| **FRI DAY** | | |

*Progress Not Perfection!*

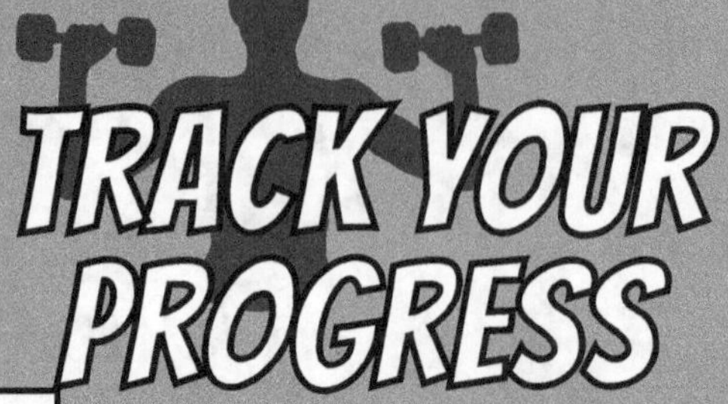


Date:_____________________

|  | EXERCISE | GOAL |
|---|---|---|
| **MON DAY** | | |
| **TUES DAY** | | |
| **WEDNES DAY** | | |
| **THURS DAY** | | |
| **FRI DAY** | | |

*Progress Not Perfection!*

# TRACK YOUR PROGRESS

Date:_________________________

| | EXERCISE | GOAL |
|---|---|---|
| **MON DAY** | | |
| **TUES DAY** | | |
| **WEDNES DAY** | | |
| **THURS DAY** | | |
| **FRI DAY** | | |

*Progress Not Perfection!*

# TRACK YOUR PROGRESS

Date:_____________________

| | EXERCISE | GOAL |
|---|---|---|
| **MON DAY** | | |
| **TUES DAY** | | |
| **WEDNES DAY** | | |
| **THURS DAY** | | |
| **FRI DAY** | | |

*Progress Not Perfection!*

www.ingramcontent.com/pod-product-compliance
Lightning Source LLC
Chambersburg PA
CBHW070913260726
48661CB00004B/1716